SOME
LIVES!

SOME LIVES!

A GP'S EAST END

DAVID WIDGERY

With photographs by
SYDNEY SHELTON

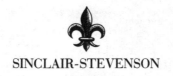

SINCLAIR-STEVENSON

To Jack and Margaret
who taught me to love London

First published in Great Britain by
Sinclair-Stevenson Limited
7/8 Kendrick Mews
London SW7 3HG, England

Copyright © 1991 by David Widgery

British Library Cataloguing in Publication Data
A CIP catalogue record for this book is available from the British Library.
ISBN: 1 85619 073 0

Phototypeset by Intype, London
Printed and bound in Great Britain by Butler & Tanner Ltd, Frome and London

ACKNOWLEDGEMENTS

With thanks to my colleagues at Gill Street for their tolerance, my patients for their good humour and Jenny Overton, Ed Emery and Ana Ransom for their work on the manuscript. The identities of all persons mentioned within the book have been altered to preserve confidentiality. The views expressed in this book are those of myself alone.

'There is no district in London with a higher proportion of decent law-abiding workers, kind-hearted, philosophical and humorous: of hard-working mothers, hanging out their flags of victory on the weekly clothes line: or so many laughing, charming, devil-may-care children, risking their lives among the traffic of Commercial Road, playing perilously about canal barges, playing sporting cricket in the streets, or gathering firewood on the Thames foreshore. Baffling youngsters – some lights, some limbs!'

Reverend Birch of St Anne's Limehouse, 1930

CONTENTS

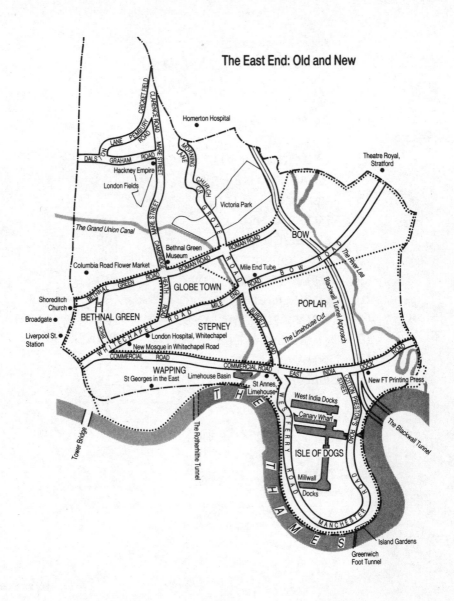

The East End: Old and New

CHAPTER 1

⊃○◉○⊂

ON YER BUS

Hackney, Mare Street. Twenty past 8 on Monday morning. Rain pelting down. The road at a standstill through sheer weight of traffic; ill-tempered cars, double-banked buses and grinding HGVs. People dart dangerously between vehicles, building workers jack-in-a-box out of transits, mothers weave buggies between revving Cortinas. The terracotta muse high above the roof of the Hackney Empire waves people to work, abstractedly. Everyone in a sudden, sodden hurry. A crowd masses and mills at the bus stop outside the Central Hall. Between them lurches a woman in mauve overcoat and carpet slippers belabouring the world in torrid patois. Each outburst culminates in the repeated cadence of 'Ras Clat Cunt'. Is she psychotic or just drunk? The schoolchildren, scared for a moment, part to let her through, reverting at once to their quarrels. The rest of the queue returns its attention variously to its newspapers, Walkmen, fags and conversation. I'm still trying to get through the Sunday paper which informs me encouragingly, 'Whatever your origins or standing in the wider world, to be waiting at a bus stop in Hackney is to have joined the ranks of the underdog.'

Mare Street at the turn of the century was a prosperous shopping street. Hackney was a suburb where successful artisans and the rising lower middle classes came to live. Pevsner in *The Buildings of England* speaks of its 'former prosperity and salubrious verdure'. Its more opulent houses have room for a maid in the basement and a piano in the parlour. Indeed, it is said that piano-teaching German refugees from the repression which followed the unsuccessful revolutions of 1848 came especially to Hackney because so many parents here wanted their children to learn the piano, whose mastery was such a part of Victorian rectitude. In 1901, when the Empire Theatre of Varieties opened, electricity had only just arrived but Mare Street, newly widened with a central tram line running to the West India Docks through Victoria Park, looked, above street level at least, strikingly similar. Today its shops are a vivid mess of bargain clothes and shoe stores, doner kebab and fried chicken takeaways and Silk Cut 'n' Sun news-agents stacked high with fizzy pop and sliced bread.

Even from this bus stop you can see the signs of the modern borough's economic hardship. Down the road a desperate line of families, children tearful, queuing outside the Homeless Persons Unit, across Mare Street a jeans shop distrained and padlocked by the bailiffs, and the chilly schoolkids in their thin, ill-fitting anoraks and leaky trainers. The gloom and hardship are count-ered, as in the 1930s, with sweets and cigarettes along with booze and video, the cheap consolations of a depressing life. Litter, everywhere despite the road-sweepers' efforts, is a symbol of the general messy unplanned neglect of our city, the piled black bags housing London's lost soul. We live, I remind myself, in the only capital city in Europe which has no elected authority. Therefore a city that dare not speak its name.

Bus No. D6, an OPO (one person operated) megabus which is the modern, far slower version of the old Limehouse tram, swerves to a halt. The queue swarms aboard flapping its bus passes, a fine Hackney muddle of neat Kurds, Orthodox Jews, rowdy British-born Afro-Caribbeans, roly-poly Chinese, dour proletarians,

2

recent immigrants and distressed leftists. When it gets going there's a fairly straight run down to Well Street where the original Stavros, the kebab-house philosopher, had his restaurant on the ground floor of a once grand late Victorian terrace. The bus judders past the Frampton Park Estate which is covered with a scaffold and polythene toupee, while its notoriously leaky roofs are at long last repaired. Strange the municipal mentality which thought all you had to do with housing was build it and the maintenance and repair would mysteriously look after itself; even the Ritz would be a slum in a fortnight if it wasn't looked after. And in the bad old days there were at least caretakers who lived on each estate rather than mobile vans which now nose around at night not very knowledgeably.

I recall being called to a patient who had died of a heart attack on the Frampton once and being surprised that the police officer on the scene was refusing the wife admission to the flat until I had certified death. In the bedroom it became obvious. The chap had died masturbating and even after a few hours' rigor mortis had his hand clamped around his still tumescent penis. The police had already tidied away the sex magazines, and after my examination we tidied him up too. 'Did he, er, achieve what he intended, Doc?' inquired the Scots policeman as I went to console the excommunicated widow. Do we ever?

The kids who occupy the front of the bus get still more noisy as they approach the impending discipline of school. 'And then he twines him and blasts the next geezer and just touches it in. Safeness' (football). 'So I just blanks him and he starts giving me licks' (psychology). 'He's a fuckin' African, so how am I supposed to understand him?!' (Afro-Caribbean boy). 'Well, if you don't understand him, how are you going to do your work?' (friend). 'That's my fuckin' excuse, man' (pedagogy). Some girls, with more grown-up manners, discuss a mutual friend. 'She had a hole. A hole in her heart, I think. They needed so much money that by the time it was raised, she was fuckin' dead.' 'How far was the sponsored walk then?' 'Oh, thirty-three miles.' Some Bengali kids are having a heated argument, in the middle of which odd Cockney phrases and Anglo-Saxon swearwords pop up. Ten-year-olds bellow profanities like troopers. Yesterday a health visitor at work was greeted by a four-year-old with the words 'Fuckin' wog'.

We're approaching Bethnal Green and the shops get still more seedy. This was the premier slum area of East London in the nineteenth century looming large in the early social reports of Chadwick and Southwood Smith and the poverty mapped by Charles Booth. Despite the efforts of housing reform, some of the spots earmarked by Booth, like the modern Boundary Estate site of Arthur Morrison's 'Old Jago', remain desperately poor. We pass a cinema turned snooker club, now closed; then a small one-time printshop which has been a suntan parlour, a tyre centre and now sells security equipment, all in the course of three years. A half-rebuilt Chinese takeaway on which work has halted. An 'antique shop' whose owner can't spell 'clearance'. And Mrs Greer, dear old Mrs 'High Class Confectionery' Greer, who remembers the Mosley days and always puts a strike collection box on her newsagents counter. Hump, over the canal bridge. On top of the map the council erected to explain the history of this branch of the Grand Union Canal (which links the Thames to the Midlands and was a significant commercial route until the Second World War), someone has painstakingly scratched an arrow and added the instruction 'Fuck here'. On the front of the bus is a London Transport poster which announces 'Graffiti is Vandalism'. I think it goes on to say 'Vandalism is Crime'. But it has been vandalised.

When I first arrived in Bethnal Green nearly twenty years ago, it was by an alphabetical accident. The dean of my medical school, the Royal Free, then in Gray's Inn Road, had decided to reward my insubordination

and lassitude by exiling me to do house jobs in Shrews-
bury. Instead I went through the London telephone
directory's list of hospitals to solicit for alternatives.
Bethnal Green Hospital, then a thriving and busy general hospital, was first in the phone book and its hospital
secretary, a kindly ex-RAF man with a walrus mous-
tache, told me over the phone to hop into a taxi, interviews were being held that morning. Although a Londoner, my knowledge of the east was distinctly sketchy.
After lodging in King's Cross for several years, I can
remember pushing my pedal bike up to the summit of
Pentonville Road, on my way to an accommodation
agency run mainly for West Indians by a Jewish couple
on a trestle table, cash-only basis, above the Angel
Electricity showrooms. Well, now I'm really in the East
End, I thought as I scaled N1. On my way down the
derelict Hackney Road to the interview at Bethnal
Green Hospital, the cab driver sensed apprehension.
'Rough diamonds,' he muttered several times. 'They
can cut up a bit when they've had a few. But if you
ever get any trouble in Casualty, you just hail a black
cab and one of our lads will sort it out for you.'

Trouble there certainly was: Casualty at Bethnal
Green frequently ended up as a mêlée of blood, sutures
and plaster of paris footprints. I was frightened for most
of my first year as a doctor. But taxi drivers there
were not. Not even when I wanted a ride home after a
weekend on duty; far less to intervene in punch-ups.
Now the fine old hospital, in which I lived for a year
as a house officer, is empty and on the market for its
land value. But whenever I pass it, I remember the
exhilarating four months when local people occupied
the Casualty in defiance of the closure orders. Better to
have fought and lost. . . . Now the hospital has a huge
yellow 'For Sale' hoarding outside it. But with the
slump in the property market who wants to buy a used
hospital?

The bus stops outside a pub that was the 'Arabian
Arms' when I first knew it, famous both for its drag

and the underground gents toilet at the adjacent traffic island. I remember being shocked in there, not because of the drag acts, but by the respectable working-class families in Sunday best cheering the outrageous acts on. Then the 'Arabian' got Ibizaised (and the toilet was filled in) and it was all strobe lights and mirrors, a modern gin palace open all hours, part of a little mid-1980s night-life renaissance in the Hackney Road. When that went phut the decor went through a Thai and cocktails period, and then became a disco again. The lunchtime strippers continued throughout. Now it's transmogrified into 'Metropolis' with a rather sinister silvery metallic female singer with a Grace Jones haircut mounted over the entrance. Still at least it's not boarded up, like so many East End pubs are in the 1990s.

Then past the pompous Edwardian-baroque town hall in Patriot Square, redolent of East London loyal and lousy. I remember the civic reception here for John H. Stracey, the Bethnal Green welterweight who briefly held the world title. Springing to the top of the steps, he cracked out of the side of his lantern jaw, 'Only ever come here before for me rent rebate.' Boxing bills still fill the York Hall in the Old Ford Road and in its Turkish baths steam a sometimes uneasy mixture of boxers, market traders and gay cruisers, including a tall, well-proportioned lawyer who looks like the ghost of Colin MacInnes and gives some of the wayward boys legal advice as he massages them. The upper deck is emptying now, to join the Central Line at Bethnal Green tube station, scene of the terrible crowd disaster during the Blitz. The Toy Museum sits next to Barmy Park on the left, a beautifully cantilevered branch of the V and A brought to the east to improve the plebs in 1875. Staring back at it balefully is the Medical Mission with its large lettering announcing 'Jesus says come unto me and I will give you rest'. Incongruously the other half of the building is occupied by the famous Balls Bros Wine Centre leading on to Paradise Row in which once lived Daniel Mendoza, the first Jewish heavyweight champion of the world.

For five years I worked as an assistant to an elderly Jewish GP whose surgery was high over a chemist in Bethnal Green Road. Like many East End GPs, he was a medical deviant, fiercely independent, blunt to his patients who none the less admired him and relied on his skill and industry. He and I would have long philosophical arguments about art, politics and history in the Venus Steak House in our lunch hours. He would tell me about the inherent imperfectibility of human nature and reminisce about Bethnal Green in the days of the Krays when East London was somehow more sealed off and the particular sharpness of Cockney speech had not yet been watered down into an inexpressive London-wide idiom.

'Before rehousing,' says Michael Leibson, 'in the narrow turning by my surgery there were thirty or forty terraced houses, most of them shared by two families. So it was a village within a village of about 500 people where everybody knew everybody else, what people did and didn't do. And everyone talked and gossiped and played together and looked after each other.' High-rise and high-density redevelopment stopped ten years ago but its social consequences remain.

The 'old' East End of the 1950s and early 1960s was indeed a very different world: of real pearly kings, family drag, nearly a dozen cinemas, nine general hospitals each with its own casualty department, a population much larger than the present Tower Hamlets' 166,000, most of whom had stable jobs with apprenticeships and 'nice' homes; a vast, autonomous, in some ways innocent proletarian city basking in the long economic boom. It may have had street prostitutes and 'red light' districts but little rape or child sexual abuse was reported. There were buckets of beer but no heroin, set-piece gang battles but few random muggings, and the traditional working-class family, so laboriously described by Wilmot and Young in *Family and Kinship*

7

in East London, was often intact, complete with stern father, omniscient mum, the Sunday roast, the Sunday best and no answering back.

The bus is now in Tower Hamlets, the central segment of that great corridor of working-class London which stretches from Whitechapel to Dagenham, which was then, apart from the odd priest, schoolteacher and GP, largely separate from bourgeois London. Indeed, the Isle of Dogs declared UDI in 1968 as its own riverside republic. As a scion of North London, I can still remember the shock of hitting the East End and realising how different this riverside republic was, the Blue Bridge by night with docked ocean liners in the impounded water within and the Thames scudding past outside, the dockers, hundreds of them, marching off shift through Chinatown and past 'Charlie Brown's' in the West India Dock Road in suits and Brylcreem, Queenie Watts's raucous, poignant, after-hours blues at the 'Iron Bridge', Jewish Brick Lane slowly transmogrifying into an Asian high street.

I can remember, too, the shock of making home visits to what were then called the 'dump estates' in Bethnal Green: like Newcourt House with its threatening graffiti ('Well, would you live here?' was painted on one wall), feuding neighbours and cacophony of shouting, cooking smells and laundry. Bethnal Green Estate had each block named after a figure from English literature: Swinburne, Milton, Moore, etc. Here a patient murdered his wife and then cut her up in the bathroom in Morris House. And in Keats, a social worker and I had to frogmarch a suicidal Bangladeshi mother of seven, who had set light to her own home, to the local mental hospital. Blake House was for a while the headquarters of an active fascist grouping. What fearful symmetry.

Now we're heading down the Roman Road past the old fire station taken over as a Buddhist meditation centre and spawning a little quarter of bookshops, design workshops and a vegetarian restaurant full of

8

arch social workers. The Roman Road shops remain white working-class smart: tropical fish, ladies' suits, wedding Rolls-Royces and lingerie boutiques. With a lot of 'lease for sale' signs. Many shoppers are Cockneys who have migrated out to Essex but who can't stay away. The bus picks up speed southwards down in the direction of the Isle of Dogs where the Canary Wharf skyscraper is half hidden in low cloud. I pass a council flat where I was called out one Easter as an emergency. It was the first contact with his doctor for fourteen years, made by an ex-docker who lived on his own. 'Fags help unclog me a bit, Doc. You will have to speak up, I'm a bit mutton.' On examination he was grossly emaciated, had a collapsed lung, a knobbly enlarged liver and about three weeks to live. His apologetic face will always stick in my mind. 'Didn't want to be a nuisance, Doc,' he insisted. 'Don't want to be a trouble.' His medical notes were still in the brown cardboard envelopes which date back to 1911 and Lloyd George with only a few faded entries in copperplate and the dog Latin the old GPs used to use. He'd had a quinsy in 1948 and a letter from the London Jewish Hospital (ADVance 1234) prescribing camphor and nasal washouts in 1952. The London Jewish, a busy Stepney general hospital built principally with moneys raised within the Jewish community but open to Gentiles, was closed in 1986 as 'surplus to requirements'. Then, to add insult to injury, it was promptly converted into a private hospital. The docks of course were all closed too by 1980, with, looking back on it, startling rapidity. My patient, a small man, had once had to scrabble hard to get the token which guaranteed a day's work. It seemed inconceivable that his brittle, shrunken, emaciated frame could have manhandled the paper sacks of cement or humped banana crates. Jack Dash, the leader of the unofficial dock shop stewards, died in the same month. He had lived to the last in Poplar, an alert presence even from his tower block. He wrote his autobiography, an elegy for the London Docks, on his kitchen table with a thick felt pen on big ruled pages. And took as his epitaph 'Here lies Jack Dash/All he wanted was/To separate them from their cash'.

When I first went to work in Limehouse, in the heart of the old docks area, I replaced a much-loved GP who had practised off the Commercial Road for forty years. I had to shake hands about twenty times a day for six months. The hands were the biggest hands I have known (even dockers' daughters have big hands). Yet a docker is now an extinct species in the East End whom I meet only when they are dying. Big sprawling men beached by illness, bluff but petrified inside, their wives crying quietly in the kitchen while pretending to make a white-bread sandwich neither will be able to swallow. And what do their children do? If boys, work for BT or the Post Office. Others have become messenger 'boys' in the City, cheerfully delivering sealed packets from banking house to banking house, or adept at navigating the back steps of the Bank of England. In the early evening they sit in groups with their pints watching the young traders swig their champagne like Tizer. One or two do make it in the City in marine insurance or the trading rooms. When they come in for their travel jabs for long-haul holidays in the Seychelles or Rio, you realise with a shock who their parents are. Their daughters probably have more chance: they can be nurses, hairdressers, or secretaries (banks don't need so many people nowadays and seem to want better GCSEs than are routinely attained in East London schools). But it's arbitrary because they might equally well be on a 'scheme' or a UB40, or already in trouble with the police. The laws of a reasonably regulated capitalism ought to give people something like what they deserve; money should have some relation to merit or industry, there ought to be some sort of idea of social or public good whose best organisation is the subject of proper public debate. This was at least the view of the nineteenth-century capitalists who caused the building of so many of the public buildings of East

London: the town halls, seamen's hostels, libraries and churches.

The workers ought to know their place. But they had a place. If it was inevitable and proper that most of them were to be poor, they should not be ignorant. But now something, a conceptual cuckoo called Docklands, has come to squat in Tower Hamlets and a marketing man's projection, all façade and PR, has edged out a local economy that once worked. And sent it splattering to the ground. 'Watch out, the big money is moving in,' says a community mural on the Manchester Road just before the Blue Bridge, through which the ocean liners of the world's oceans used to edge into the great Port of London. I recall another forlorn face, an ex-engineer whose council home for twenty years will need to be demolished in order to drive the new Docklands motorway across the neck of the Isle of Dogs. We were talking in his front doorway, he in Viyella pyjamas, gaunt, each breath an effort of cough and sputum, me anxious to get home. Twenty feet away, a vast, illuminated twenty-four-hour pile driver thumped away and behind it glinted the vast greenhouse of girders which is to be the Canary Wharf complex, completely overshadowing his once quiet estate. He didn't mind the noise, he said. It was nothing if you were used to engineering factories. But didn't like them just coming into his back garden with hardly a word. 'The tenants' association has had a meeting. What can you do against John Laing and Mowlem?'

Not a lot. We've arrived at the Isle of Dogs, and although it's still early in the morning the road already has a muddy sheen from the spillage from the incessant lorries which cart earth and debris out of the vast building site. Perhaps it's what the economists call the trickle-down effect. Crossing the A13's permanent log jam, the limousines and carphonies are already sweeping down West India Dock Road to their new playground. I wait to cross outside no. 5, an old clothing manufacturer's awaiting demolition. Its window glass

11

is embossed 'Overalls, Seamen's Clothing, Fancy Goods' and in the barred doorway there is a list: 'We specialise in officers' uniforms, sea boots, donkey coats, belts and braces, hats and caps.' Over the road was the Peking Restaurant with its deep brown interior, sleepy dogs and fish tanks, now demolished. The Cantonese family that ran it for forty years, all three generations, used to argue and play cards with the cook in the back room when business was slack. It possessed a gentle, timeless air, a telephone cabinet of brown wood and a gents toilet identified with a picture of top hat, cane and silk scarf. One week it just closed without a chance to say goodbye. The family were fobbed off with premises on a blank bleak stretch of the Commercial Road where they quickly went bust. Just down from them, 'Charlie Brown's', the famous seamen's pub which used to keep a menagerie of exotic animals the sailors would hock for drink, was demolished along with 300 homes on St Vincent's Estate to make way for a new motorway to link Canary Wharf with the City.

Behind it, the vast structure of Canary Wharf is now completed, 'the greatest office development in the world' the posters say, a gigantic Beaux-Arts skyscraper in the style of 1920s-Manhattan-meets-Croydon with brass knobs supervised by Roy Strong, a pseudo-suburban centrepiece to a shambles of ill-matched, temporary-looking commercial buildings recently erected on the Isle of Dogs like so many exhibition stands. Which will one day maybe provide some local jobs as shelf-fillers and security guards.

As a sweetener from the London Docklands Development Corporation (LDDC), some of the council blocks out of the direct line of fire are being upgraded. And Hawksmoor's St Anne's Limehouse has almost finished an external refurbishment to which the corporation has also contributed. The church was one of the twelve built as a result of the over-optimistic 1711 Fifty Churches Act which, in a mixture of piety and politics, had planned a rapid expansion of High Church premises in inner London, both to celebrate the return to power of the Tories in 1710 and to counter the spread of the Dissenting chapels in the East End. It still stands with its mysterious churchyard, Solemn and Awful, the octagonal summit of its steeple constructed of columns and obelisks visible from throughout the borough, its flag once a familiar landmark to returning seamen. Once a year in its churchyard a festival is held. Everyone mucks in: the local firms give wood, scaffolding, paintbrushes and tent pegs, the OPA club makes bunting and cakes, community transport provide electricity and parking, the school's community group helps with the play centres and the urban farm, the Chinese Welfare and the Bangladeshi Youth Association all contribute. In a kind of way it's a more secular parallel of the social work undertaken by the Limehouse Church Institute. For an afternoon Limehouse is a village, although it's hard to completely ignore the thundering of the A13 traffic which grinds incessantly past the churchyard.

The Limehouse Church Institute was adjacent to St Anne's, opened in 1904 by the Bishop of London as a centre for community and educational activities. In 1912 there was a gymnastic club, a branch of the Church of England's Men's Society, a church lads' brigade, a mothers' meeting place and a missionary association. It is still remembered fondly by older Limehouse residents as a much-loved centre of community support and for those in social need. Typically, it has been converted to luxury housing which in the housing slump remains unoccupied. Many locals signed a petition, bound to be ignored given the virtual suspension of planning law within Docklands, against its conversion. The developers' highly unreal brochure is ecstatic about what lies 'behind a handsome listed façade' including 'hand-painted fitted wardrobes', 'tiled terraces, Magnificent Main Entrance and Common Parts' and 'TV Points Adaptable to Sky TV'. The brochure attempts to transcend the semi-permanent traffic jam by a montage of

13

the short-takeoff planes at the City Airport, the Thames Line river bus and the gentlemen windsurfing in Millwall Dock with, for some reason, the Post Office Tower stuck above it. From the berths and cargo sheds of empire to the shopping malls of suburbia. From the church lads' brigade and the missionary society to Sky TV and fitted wardrobes. Only the slump in property prices was so steep in Docklands that the developers now prefer to lease the flats to the council to house homeless families. So maybe the market isn't so bad after all?

Perhaps we shouldn't complain. Our health centre, the first to open in Tower Hamlets but now showing its age, has been rebuilt too, with majority finance from the LDDC. But then so it should be. The reality, behind the handsome façade of estate agentese, of the area immediately around St Anne's Limehouse is grim and, despite Docklands, getting grimmer. The patients are often ill-fed and ill-housed as well as plain ill.

The real unemployment rate is 30 per cent or above and rising more sharply now as it did in the early 1980s, it has one of the highest morbidity and GP consultation rates in Britain and a high turnover rate which is accelerated by the high proportion of hostel dwellers including those in the Salvation Army single men's hostel detoxification unit in Garford Street, the Copenhagen Place alcoholics hostel and the Tower Hamlets Women's Refuge, as well as Princes Lodge which used to house the mobile unemployed adults from all over Britain. There is also an unusually high proportion of immigrants, particularly those of Chinese, Bangladeshi, Vietnamese and, most recently, Somalian origins, and bad housing stock often in an advanced state of decay, with 25 per cent technical overcrowding. The usual indicators of poverty, including car ownership and phone ownership, reflect an exceptionally poor population. There is a 30 per cent illegitimacy rate and a very high rate of single parents. None the less the fertility rate is exceptionally high (GFR 10 per cent above the North

Thames average and 40 per cent above the national average).

Although not obvious to the casual observer, St Vincent's Estate in particular has a very large number of under-five-year-old children, yet the area is dominated by heavy traffic from the construction sites and there is very little access to open or safe playspace. Poplar Play Centre has a waiting list of 180 children. The district psychologist for Tower Hamlets told the Tower Hamlets Health Authority Inquiry last year, 'Tower Hamlets is a particularly difficult place to bring up small children: the large number of high-rise blocks, the lack of gardens, the lack of safe spaces for mothers and children to play really makes the whole child-rearing period very difficult.' Or the different London boroughs in which she had worked: 'The degree of isolation, depression and child behavioural problems are really the worst I have seen anywhere.'

But what we get is NHS cuts, penthouses, poll tax and Canary Wharf. And this little sequence of Limehouse events is being repeated all over the East End, especially anywhere with a view of water. It is, I reflect, plodding through the muddy puddles of the building work, a microcosm, a rather large microcosm, of what happened to Britain in the 1980s.

It is possible to describe this process in many ways. As the product of political economy and the way the City and deregulated finance capital have triumphed over manufacture to such a degree in late twentieth-century Britain. Or as a geopolitical imperative, impossible to halt and ludicrous to oppose, by which water transport and the industries and skills required to sustain it have been vanquished by road and air transport. It could even be seen (if you were to close your eyes almost completely and believe in the façade, and there are nowadays plenty of thirty-year-olds who seem to do this successfully) as part of a great leap forward to freedom (redefined as the market) against all the unwanted nonsense of the Welfare State and comprehensive education and council housing and municipal socialism.

I have come to see the process more intimately and more personally. Partly it is what has happened to me, the grinding down of the optimism with which I came as a doctor to the East End nearly twenty years ago, into a kind of grudging weariness punctuated with bouts of petty fury. When I came here in that fateful taxi down Hackney Road, I didn't know what the bruised face of a raped heroin addict was like, or how children could be locked up without food, four in a room, by a drunken father as a punishment, or what happens to a jaw when it is broken in a domestic fight and concealed. And now I do. I know what decomposed bodies of alcoholics smell like after two weeks, and the noises made when dying in pain, and what happens to a woman's face when she is told her breast cancer has spread. I think I wish I didn't.

Perhaps this would have happened anywhere as part of the process of growing up, medically and personally. But more importantly, my experience reflects a much larger loss of hope, morale and optimism among those who live in the East End. In the young it's expressed in a kind of nihilism which is impossible sometimes to penetrate. In the old it's more often a nostalgia. It is a yearning for a now gone world of urban optimism and rising working-class quality of life. And a memory of a sense of solidarity, built through the unions and forged in the Blitz, a trust and a unity which are worth a great deal more than a share in Thames Water or a fly-drive holiday in Nevada. It is also a bitterness, now widely and rightly felt in East London, that far from benefiting from the movement of big capital into the area, locals are being undermined and impoverished by docklands redevelopment.

I'm watching something die and I wish I wasn't. Perhaps the best that can be done is to record the process.

16

CHAPTER 2

EPIPHANIES

Jamaican. Devout mother in neat Sunday bonnet and perm with mute choirboy son who is probably schizophrenic. She says he won't talk because 'Mad Irish nurse tried to shake the evil into him'. The East End is like Amsterdam one moment, Harlem the next. The Pentecostals eat bagels in Ridley Road after their limbo-trance in Nuttall Street.

A note under the surgery door:

> MR AND MRS FREDERICK SAPOSNIK
> CRAMPS TOP LEG.
> FAINTED. JUST HAD HEART TROUBLE.
> JOB TO BREATHE.
> ENARD HOUSE.

No request for haste in the letter but I hurry round. Mr Saposnik's dying; Mrs S. offers tea. Despite two coronary bypasses, he's now strangled with anoxic pain, face grey, clutching for throat. We wait for the ambulance, window open to identify us, her doilies neatly heaped on the local paper, the cat perturbed by me frantically resuscitating. 'Come,' she used to say, 'as long as you don't think he's wasting your time.' That reflex in an old 'un, prepared to make a tactical

17

retreat but also courtesy. To advance with charm or a curse. He is dead now. The ambulance hasn't come.

'Now don't let me see you do that again.'
    'I said don't do that again and I meant it.'
    'I said sit on the chair and I *meant* it.'
    Father looks up from drinking Special Brew. 'Your mother doesn't let you do that.' The boy is speech-delayed and disinhibited.
    'Could you kindly come and see the boy. I was Dr Teverson's patient. He used to call here. I cannot come to see you. I'm having a bit of trouble with the child.' The child is twenty-eight years old.

Past the amputee in Guinness Buildings, the stroke in Benn House, the nutty whites who say they are being poisoned and the blacks fearful of them. What can you tell from how a door opens to you: whether it is left ajar or needs complex unbolting? Chains clatter.
    'I've been very aggravated in myself. Give me a good examination.'
    'Where's your daughter?'
    'She lives in Chigwell,' with an especially weary tone. 'Anyhow,' with that nightcleaner's sigh, 'I've had a couple.' She means a bottle. It's lunchtime. She shows me a lawyer's letter: 'I understand she lived with a man for seven years until four years ago and she describes being "tricked" by him into believing they would eventually marry and have children but in the end he left to have children with somebody else.' Then she shows her breast. 'It's just a festered pimple.' It's an ulcerated carcinoma of the breast, indurated, probably inoperable. As she covers up, she grimaces; 'I don't envy you young 'uns.' 'We've lost a lot, what people don't realise.' She will take her time to die; the ulcerated ones are indolent.

I would be very grateful if you would call on my grand-mother. Her legs and feet are very swollen and she cannot walk at all. Also, her eyesight is failing with another cataract. I am very frightened that she is going to have a terrible accident, as there is nobody with her and I am living in Essex.

She is Irish. 'Don't know anything about Ireland? You must live in England,' she says when I ask about Donegal. 'Bugs in the bed, although I'm one of those people who has always been hygienic.' There has been trouble down at the Social. They won't pay her benefit any more.

She's one of those many East Enders who find it impossible to pronounce the word 'certificate' properly.

'Well, see you later, another day, maybe tomorrow.'

Her smiles are well-composed masks, little snatches of decency. 'I'll try leaving off greens which don't please me.'

GPs are like publicans, they too have to manufacture smiles and remember the names of their regulars.

Lady smiles benignly at her sepia wedding photos. 'To be quite honest I'm bored silly with my job; do frozen dinners for the caravan, talk about our last holiday, the kids have left home.' She talks of the past: when streets were little theatres, pubs gleamed, faces were big, peering up to life's lens, magnified by the quirkiness of memory. They were her coster uncles up the Lane: gargoyle faces under flat caps selling novelties with jolly eyes in tunnels slippery with squashed fruit.

Now continental lorry drivers sit in 'The Ten Bells'. It was briefly called 'The Jack the Ripper' but Feminists Against Male Violence objected. Two prostitutes come in and start working the bar. There is now a special HIV clinic for street workers at the Royal London Hospital, 'street workers' being people who sell sex but don't define themselves as prostitutes. The joys of nomenclature. A Muslim chef in a white cap is complaining to the suppliers on his mobile phone about the condition

19

of his chickens which sit, broken-necked, in a crate on the pavement of Brick Lane. Businessmen eat curried fish with rosé in Hanbury Street. In the window of B. Weinburg Printer are cards for Minsky (Furs), London, Manchester and Bradford, Elegante Fashions, Berwick Street. Labovitch the Glazier becomes David Glassman and family, Woodford Green. The new police station radiates an unearthly blue gleam.

'Fuk off Wogs' is scratched in the doorway.

'You cannot ask how I am. Only how life is treating me,' says Markovitch. He got a pop-up toaster for his leaving present. After thirty years.

'My married life, sometimes I just want to scream. I'm sick of just the view over the desk. Ugh.'

This column has been provided for doctors to enter A, V or C at their discretion.

'I wanted to holler,' says Markovitch. 'And one more thing. About the grandchild. It needs a check-up. I'm a great believer in salt myself. I have to have it because it draws. Haven't been outside that door for weeks.'

From the surgery window I watch the cortège of Jade Nessa edge down Bethnal Green Road. A seven-year-old made wisp-like with leukaemia, kept alive by the intensity of her smile, it sometimes seemed. A union of Dacca and E2, fending off death most of her life. Blasted with cytotoxics, vomiting and needle-bruised, I saw her just before she died, and she made her will, smiling to me. 'I want Ivan (the boy next door) to have my bike.' The bike, unridden for three years, leant against the wall beside us. 'And the cuddlies will go to the kids at the hospital.' Few adults can be so brave. On the main floral display it says: 'In the end she died so quietly.' People weep in the street in front of the funeral's louche exhibitionism. Press the bell for the next patients: ted with tattoos and bronchitis, gay with a stiff neck, depressed book-keeper, fed-up West Indian, boy with conker allergy, stiff-backed lorry driver. Old dear just out of hospital: 'Downstairs it was nice but upstairs it was them geriatrics. I'll see you, Doc, bye bye.' Life goes on.

> Dear Doctor During my period it is only Bleeding very little. So please kindly give some tablet or medicine to bleed properly. Mrs Begum.

'I want to choke them and poison them and shake the place to pieces.' Mr Svensen.

'No jobs!' Svensen shouts. 'I was made redundant, wasn't I!'

'It's his stomach, you know,' says Mrs Svensen. Pause, meaningful. 'It aggravates. He was aggravated by the inspector. Business is slack so they'll use the least excuse. People will give a lot for a job these days.'

'Mustn't grumble,' says Svensen. 'Only got mugged, didn't I. Beer with friends, money stole, didn't see his face. They grab hold of things. We don't have the right to be considered. But my stamps are in order.'

'Got the touch of a flu,' says old Jenny Crudgington. 'I came all over like a reeling drunken man although I am a total abstainer.

'Hold on to your corsets, Jenny,' I said to myself.

'Come about my water. I mean my daughter.'

'Schools. First you lose the milk then you lose the meals.'

'I love babies, that's my trouble,' says chirpy Thelma Korbel smiling at the squalor. The baby squalls. Grandad went to America, the home of advanced ideas; the electric chair, deforestation, baked beans. He sent money 'for you poor East End Jews'. Sticker in the lift: 'What's the difference between niggers and gorillas? Gorillas better looking.'

Neurotic Naomi, her mother, orchestrates the cleaning ladies on the 22 to complain about feckless families, to write imaginary letters, which she recites to the entire lower deck, to the housing, the bank, the boss, about the dogs, the neighbours, the coppers. To the slimming club about the psychologist and the probation office about the fish and chips under her pillow which stop her sleeping at night.

Thelma and Naomi. 'Don't be a baby, Thelma. I love Thelma's children too. She's a delicate child. She wants to be a driving instructor. She buys cheap jewellery and fantasy wigs in Zeids. Another bloody pair of high heels, I used to say. Heels!' What colour, how much, how long? Endless interrogation of Thelma before I am allowed to inquire, 'Your vulva, is it sore, tender or irritated?'

Thelma's turn now. 'The lump comes up like a little lump of fire. I think I'm allergic to sanitary towels. I've got the giddy fever. Everyone I know has taken a liking to you. But I'm Thelma. I'm one that won't give in.'

The two of them wave goodbye in unison, as if animated, their neuroticism coiled and polished. The baby squalls. Poor baby.

Evening surgery: note entries shorten, examinations perfunctory or postponed, tempers fray.

'He's so bad with money.'

'They break their bones fighting over a woman.'

'So what!'

'Well, she has opinions on most things now. She clung to me and said, "Postpone it."'

'Death I think she meant. She knew she was going to die. Then she starts rambling. She says she wants my money. Or I want hers.'

'Sometimes I get right fed up. We're getting too old. I wish I could live properly.'

Oh, get on with it. Very last patient, queuing in the waiting room holding back tears, lips raw with biting and with pain. 'I didn't let on. Well, I knew about the pain. It was at night when it came. He wouldn't let on.' She was widowed two days ago. Well, there's not much I can do.

Then home visits: 'Little Tracey's never wanted for

anything. Tracey, the bogey man will get you, hands off I tell you, or Doctor will stick a needle into you.' Incontinent of course.

Disaster rides shotgun in the happy family, you've already been warned. Then a postnatal infection. Cluster of needle-headed boils on the perineum. But more importantly, Ruth Baxter is attempting to execute her baby: full-scale puerperal psychosis. 'When it rears its ugly head it goes straight to my stomach,' she says as I examine. When her husband's not looking she tries to throw the baby out of the window. Like Punch and Judy. Puerperal psychosis: 'a psychiatric emergency'. But so are all of them; cramped flats, every inch of space occupied, beds a battlefield, stairs lethal. Calls for drinks, calls for food, clothes to be found, children to be silenced, arguments about plans. Nobody agrees. Dad shouts. Mum cries. The children go silent. Ruth is florid. So she gets ECT.

Mrs Lee has Alzheimer's: 'David, I can't tell you the pain I'm in.'

'Your husband tells me you are out a lot.'

'Well, he's a born liar. Can't live on pension. Don't know who to talk to. Kids herd me about.'

I speak to her husband separately: 'My time with her is twenty-four hours a day. You know yourself as a doctor that it's not the right thing to be swearing so. She's a married woman.'

Mrs Lee: 'I don't have time for love and all that business. At hospital I never see the same doctor. At home I just look at the dustbins. And everybody looks at me.' She was the first white woman in Bethnal Green to marry a Chinaman. She is still a beauty.

'Well, bye bye, sweetheart.'

'Well are you going to be all right, Mrs Lee?'

'David, I can't complain. I'm upright and I've got my family.'

We part with a well-timed volley of her coughs.

Mrs Veitch, a strong woman, folds hands by sink. 'You'd better go and look at him.' He is tucked up in a bed firmly like a wedge of cheese. A railway porter at Liverpool Street with a far-away look in his eyes. Once he had told me, 'We're the working class and we'll never alter.' He has a darting toothy grin.

His death came on Good Friday in a room full of boxing photos. I was there.

He said just before he died, 'You've been a good wife.'

She said, 'Let's not talk like that.'

She says afterwards, 'He went quiet. But he was big. I did me back lifting him.'

She has a letter from her son:

Dear Mum
I hope you are well and happy. Thank you for your letter. I was glad to hear that you got home alright even though you did go the long way round. I got a letter from Bill and he also sent me £5 to buy papers. He said he was glad to hear I only got four years. I am growing a beard because I am fed up with shaving all the time but have come out in a rash. Prison isn't so bad. Sorry to hear about Dad.

Used to have the emergency care of a left-wing printshop: urgent visas, nervous breakdowns from nothing more sinister than overwork, asthma pumps for people who spent too much time in the pub to go to the doctor, back pain that 'surely should have resolved by now'. Nice people, plucky, doing something they believed in within a hectic ideological framework, often kind to each other and concerned with quite normal things: football leagues and works outings. Not the old queue and shufflers at the sick-shop: 'I won't be delaying you, you've got quite a crowd', 'If you're not ill when you come here, you're ill when you leave', 'Now listen, Doctor, I don't know if it's nothing or something', 'I know you are busy but . . .'

'Something to sleep me at night?'

'Cheers,' says Mr Patel.

WE WANT MORE MONEY FOR THE NHS BUT TO
RAISE IT BY INCREASING PRESCRIPTION CHARGES
IS TO PUT A TAX ON THE SICK WHO CAN LEAST
AFFORD IT. IT IS TO TURN PHARMACISTS INTO
TAX COLLECTORS AND MAKE DOCTORS THINK
FIRST OF THE PATIENT'S FINANCIAL STATE,
RATHER THAN THE BEST AVAILABLE TREATMENTS.

If you agree with this leaflet please display it
and distribute it.

'My stomach's wrong. Ate something out Debden
way. Couldn't refuse. Stewed apple. Don't eat that
much apple. While I'm here, can I have a pair of elastic
stockings. Thigh-length. Lightweight. Make it two
pairs because I have to wash them.'

'Too much pain, little bit all right, here is too much.'

'My skin: it's like an army of ants.'

A woman of fifty says, 'I've got Daddy outside with
ear trouble.'

He says, 'Playing me up now worse than ever.'

'Wish you luck,' says an indecent exposer. 'You're
not after a young lady, are you?'

'Can I see a professor in blood pressure?' I tell him I
am one.

'Lovely sleep, but woke up screaming in a terrible fight.
Oh my Billy. Gas meter broken in again, the holy
terrors. If I don't give them the money, they steal. And
when I'm pregnant they trade off it.

'Billy, he needs shooting; if you hear a big bang you
will know I've succeeded.'

Billy says, 'Had a bit of a nervous breakdown last
week. Went up St Clement's. Now I'm dosed up to
the hilt. So I can't change my underclothes.'

Sits in tiny kitchen with heat on. 'I go to bed with

the shakes and get up with the shakes. Makes me feel ancient.'

Billy is transvestite; eye liner running, legs wrong, far too much thigh. Up the pub usually. Later he burns to death.

Indian lad peeks round the door with Coke can and flu. See old Elizabeth Smith, huge Rembrandt eyes, who manages to grow wisteria out of big catering pea tins on the landing. But Annie the Pill gets me on the stairs: 'Pills pills PAIN PAIN. Hallo, old Widggey, remember me, I'm the Codeine Girl. You can't eat the yolk before the egg: that's an old Jewish saying.'

'You have to come to surgery.'

'You bastard.' She snarls. I must tell the Royal College of General Practitioners Prescribing Sub-Committee about her.

Elizabeth Smith puts head back round the door. 'Have you got a wife? She must be very patient.'

Punks with their dogs piss in the waiting room and ask for money. Saul the furrier is depressed again. When he's depressed, he stutters. 'I think it's a sin to answer a doctor back,' he says. Because he's angry and wants to shout at me, at anyone. But can't.

I tell him in a depression manners are the first casualties. 'Are you drinking, Saul?'

'One Guinness since Christmas. It's God's truth!'

Saul's wife's fed up. 'I was a lovely woman and kept myself clean.

'Now I'm short of breath and couldn't hardly breathe.'

Saul doesn't like the question. 'I do know but to explain would take half an hour. Oh, it's a shithole like everywhere else.' He gets a few drinks and wants to wipe everybody out.

'When you feel happy you can share happiness, but we never are. I tell you straight it's useless. Pills. Don't even tell me what they are.'

Mr Mercer has myeloma: 'It's a disease I can recommend to anyone.'

'He's the kind that won't give in,' says his wife. That means he's involved in an outrageous painful denial.

He's of the old school but a little Chinese girl saved his life.

He takes his terminal care in the pub: 'Can you make that a large one, Ben, the other one went too quickly.'

He died on Christmas Eve and they didn't come for the body till the day after Boxing Day. I got an engraved beer mug from the family some years later.

'Wotcha got this hammer for then?'

'It's not, it's a stethoscope. How's your chest?'

'Sounds like someone's playing the flute down there at night.

'I want to go to Bethnal Green Hospital.'

'Well, it's closed.'

He knows the sadness of a hospital closure: loss of wards he knows, familiar faces, accumulated warmth. The manager says everyone loves a hospital that's to be closed. The manager will never know why. The manager will go on somewhere else next year.

'Just stick me some Valium on there, will you. I hope you never have to take them.

'I wake up and I'm all pain in the tubes.'

His wife calls me that night. 'Quick. Now put your coat on and come quick. He's faintified and sickified.'

He's cyanosed, hyperventilating. It's not worth getting out the peak flow meter.

'It's a bit dicky, like. Could you give it a once-over? Maybe I will go in. As long as you don't make me a geriatric case, Doc.'

I spend a long time with the Emergency Bed Service on the neighbour's phone. They can't get hold of the Medical Referee. 'No beds anywhere, sir.' The 'sir' is supposed to make me feel better.

SOME LIVES!

He dies in the ambulance, on the way to a hospital that isn't closed.

CHAPTER 3

---~∘⊙∘~---

IN SEARCH OF THE COCKNEY

Defining the East End is a contentious business. To be born within the sound of Bow Bells (St Mary le Bow in Cheapside not the church on the traffic island by the Bow flyover) is nowadays nearly impossible; there are few home deliveries in the City and the maternity unit at St Bart's in Smithfield has been closed. Cockney, as applied by the establishment literati to unconventional poets like Keats, means simply misshapen egg. The 'old' East End was compact, stretching from Jewish Whitechapel through Stepney to the Poplar docks: a long-gone world of intimate terraces, Yiddisher mummas and brawling stevedores. Most East Enders themselves would include Bow, Bethnal Green and Hoxton to the north and at least part of Newham to the east. Quite where East London cedes to North London is difficult to decide: usually the line of the ancient northbound Kingsland Road which slices north from the city through Hackney and Stoke Newington is taken as the dividing line. The border is still more difficult to define in the east where a long working-class residential corridor stretches through Stratford and Barking out to Dagenham and Cockney Essex.

EastEnders opens with an aerial photograph which spirals down into the Poplar heartland, the triangle formed above the Isle of Dogs between the docks, the Limehouse Cut, built in 1770, and the River Lea. But Dick Hobbs, the best sociological writer on modern East London, prefers the idea of 'a class frontier encasing a vast working-class city of the three London boroughs (Hackney, Tower Hamlets and Newham) which also influences a large part of the county of Essex'. This would describe a largely self-sufficient proletarian metropolis with a population of over 3 million souls speaking nearly 150 languages, an unequal triangle marked in the north by the Orthodox Jewish enclave in Stamford Hill, in the west by the now largely Bangladeshi Brick Lane area of Spitalfields, cheek and jowl with the City, and extending, well, as far as Rayleigh, Stanford le Hope, Brentwood and the nether regions where the Upminster Kid, Billericay Dicky and Harold Hill of Harold Hill roam through the countryside in their personalised Cortinas. I live in Hackney, work in Tower Hamlets and dislike Essex's drab loutishness so this account, like the *EastEnders* title, focuses on the central section of Tower Hamlets: the old East End boroughs of Bethnal Green, Bow and Limehouse in each of which I have practised as a doctor, for nearly twenty years.

Settlements existed in all three places in the late middle ages when the rest of what is now East London was farming and monastic land. An eighteenth-century map still showing most of present day Tower Hamlets as grazing land would register Limehouse as an independent village with its indigenous trades of lime-burning and brewing as well as its maritime connections. Bow would have shown up as a busy waterside village on the main crossing of the River Lea. And Bethnal Green was already a distinctive neighbourhood of weavers, dyers and shoe- and boot-makers. The best way to understand the East End's social geography is to appreciate that it has always been an assemblage of very diverse ingredients. Although the relentless eastward advance of eighteenth- and nineteenth-century

industrialisation appeared superficially to have obliterated the countryside and homogenised the old village
identities, the East End was still a number of quite
different communities, shaped now by street patterns
and the passage of canals, roads and railways. There
were as marked differences within the various manufacturing areas; between, say, the highly skilled silk-
weaving and clothes-making of Spitalfields and the
mass-produced shoes and boots made in Hoxton, as
between them and the riverside districts. For the
Thames communities had their own maritime identities
as well as being part of the East End. Wapping's particular reputation for disorder derived from its combination
of sailors on shore leave, the high density of liquor
stores and its long and lucrative traditions of smuggling
and pilferage. And even before the opening of the first
enclosed docks, the Isle of Dogs and Poplar had long
experience of loading and refitting ocean-going vessels.

This mosaic-like pattern of social geography had
sharpened by the end of the nineteenth century as the
East End's population rapidly expanded. A clear
polarity emerged between the Anglo-Irish dockland and
the immigrant manufacturing areas of Whitechapel and
Stepney, an axis which still shapes the borough. And
'respectable' Bow and Globetown were separated from
the less reputable 'islands' of Wapping and the Isle of
Dogs by the sanitary clearances and railways expansion
which divided the borough along an east-west axis.
Whitechapel was, as ever, poor and dire, awaiting, as
always, 'redevelopment'.

And it was from this dense, highly variegated pattern
of working-class city life that the traditional virtues of
Cockney life – cheerfulness in adversity, informality,
warmth and a relish in the collective struggle for survival – derive. It arose, quite literally, from the streets,
the terraces in which people were born and lived and
fought and made up and cried and died. Yet in modern
East London, streets of this kind, once universal, are
now uncommon. And for a particular reason. Nowhere

31

in Britain, not even Coventry and Southampton, was subjected to such intense and systematic bombing as the East End of London during the Second World War. Nowhere was the street pattern so comprehensively obliterated. So nowhere was postwar architectural megalomania so untrammelled.

The East End of London, designated Target Area A by the Luftwaffe, was the most intensively bombed area of the capital. From September 1940 to May 1941, there were nightly raids of German bombers dropping explosive and incendiary bombs on the docks and the chemical and munition factories clustered round them. In the first raid a majestic, terrible fleet of 320 Heinkel and Dornier bombers flying three miles high above the Thames pounded an unprepared East End. Patients still tell me about that day as if it were yesterday. The Blitz destroyed or damaged 3.5 million London homes, killed 29,890 people and injured 50,497. The East Enders bore the brunt of the devastation. If surviving direct hits, they would emerge from the unsafe, insanitary shelters to face out-of-control fires, sealed-off streets, falling masonry and collapsing buildings. Many mothers and children, evacuated in the phoney war period, had, homesick, returned to unprotected homes. Domestic Anderson shelters were farcically inadequate and the authorities directed people to shallow water-logged trenches ('We must have been daft to bother,' an old seamstress remembered to me) in Victoria Park.

Although the raids were initially said by the German High Command to be limited to strategic raids against military targets, the intimate indentations between the forty-three miles of docks and the residential areas of the East End made civilian casualties inevitable, especially after the introduction of parachute mines which exploded at roof level. Unexploded bombs were a major problem; many had delay timers aimed against bomb disposal experts. The doctor brother of the GP I succeeded in Limehouse was killed in Millwall Dock when a bomb exploded while he was attending to a trapped patient. Dr Moss himself was always known to his patients behind his back as 'Mossie', a wartime reference taken from the Mosquito bomber, also known as 'Mossie' and built out of wood by ex-furniture-makers in nearby Walthamstow. To this day unexploded bombs unearthed during new building regularly require evacuation.

The patients will still tell vivid stories about those days. Of evacuation ill-planned and sometimes bungled; 400 people died in a direct hit on a school in Canning Town where they had been sheltering for three days awaiting transport which had gone to Camden Town instead. Homeless families taken to Southend by steamer from Wapping Pier, other families without homes wandering the smouldering streets. Homes which had only recently acquired electricity, gas and water, losing supplies of all three again. An ex-ARP warden sitting in a geriatric ward in Bethnal Green Hospital screwed up his face as he told me one sunny afternoon about conditions in the Tilbury mass shelter where up to 16,000 huddled each night awash with floodwater, faeces and rats; 'It made Hell look like a holiday camp, son.' The Battle of London was won here, by the Cockneys, with their astonishing bravery, self-reliance and improvisation, by working-class civilians and the rescue services. Posh London, to its own embarrassment, seldom suffered. But the cost to East London was tremendous and its effects prolonged.

A third of the Port of London Authority's warehouses were destroyed, the waterfront was flattened, landmarks were obliterated, St George's in the East, St Anne's Limehouse and the London Hospital Whitechapel were damaged and direct hits on factories produced infernos. The River Lea burned blue when a gin factory sustained a direct hit and the Thames was set alight, and barges blazed after an extensive leak of liquid sugar from a burning Silvertown. The main East London sewer outflow was breached and on 3 March 1943, 173 people, in the main mothers sheltering with their children, were asphyxiated or crushed in a crowd panic on the blacked-out steps of Bethnal Green tube station on a night when, as people sorrowfully still tell you, no bombs fell anywhere in East London. And when air attacks were resumed in 1944 by the pilotless V1 and V2 doodlebugs, it was, once again, the east of the city which took the most punishment, probably for the geographical reason that these terrifying but inaccurate weapons were launched from The Hague in the Netherlands. The first V1 exploded in Bow near the railway bridge over Grove Road on 13 June 1944. These weapons were highly effective and about 20,000 homes were damaged by them, producing heavier casualties than even the bombing waves of 1940. The explosion radiated over a quarter-mile area and the silent approach and 'automatic' delivery are still given by anxious patients as the origin of their neurosis.

As the war drew to its peak in a bloodthirsty crescendo, it was the civilians in London, Berlin, Dresden, Hiroshima and Nagasaki who filled the cemeteries (the 14 February 1945 razing of Dresden, a war crime if ever there was one, killed twelve times the total number of Londoners who had died from flying bombs in the preceding nine months). The last V2 to fall on London killed 134 people in a massive explosion in flats in Vallance Road, Bethnal Green, near the place where the Kray brothers were born. When the king drove in state through East London on VE Day, the inner and outer boroughs were ravaged. The greatest density of damage was in Tower Hamlets, notably Stepney, Wapping, Poplar, Limehouse and Silvertown. But bomb damage extended out to Barking, Dagenham and Essex. Nearly a third of the population had moved away, many never to return. The East End had been made unrecognisable. Despite the courage and stoicism of the East Enders and a communal spirit which seemed sometimes to verge on an insane gaiety, the suffering and loss permanently altered Tower Hamlets in spirit and in physical experience. The theorem is quite simple. The degree of

bomb damage related directly to the location of factories and docks. The density of postwar council housing
it made possible related, in turn, directly to the degree
of bomb damage. And so it came about that in postwar
London it was the rich who got the terraces and the
poor that got the tower blocks. What the Luftwaffe
didn't get, the developers did. By the mid-1960s,
Tower Hamlets, the heart of wartime proletarian
London, had over 90 per cent of its population living
in council housing, a far higher proportion even than
the neighbouring boroughs similar in class compo-
sition.

There is, in fact, a long and honourable tradition
of good-quality public housing in East London. The
'Housing for the Working Classes' branch of the
London County Council's Architects' Department,
established in 1889, was responsible for some solid
housing in Bethnal Green and philanthropists like Burd-
ett-Coutts. Octavia Hill and the Guinness, Peabody
and Samuel Lewis Trusts had erected extensive if drab
'modern dwellings': barrack-like but soundly constructed blocks. And the interwar GLC had a formidable record for producing imaginative and architecturally sound council housing in large volumes. It was
on this tradition of civic planning that Professor Peter
Abercrombie drew up an extensive wartime plan for
the reorganisation of the entire building pattern in
London to improve transport, dispose residential
accommodation more logically and increase park and
leisure space for ordinary Londoners. Abercrombie
recognised the East End's special claim for attention
and promised, 'The East End will at last be a worthy
place in which to live, work and play.' Although there
was to be an organised exodus to the 'New Towns',
this was to be counterbalanced by the creation of a 'new
town in the East End' centred in the 130-acre Poplar
triangle between the Thames, the Limehouse Cut and
the River Lea, in which health centres, schools and
leisure facilities were planned.

Despite the pledges, rebuilding was slow to commence. As a 'short-term' solution many homeless families were given prefabricated housing parked on levelled bomb sites, pastoral bungalows bitterly cold in winter, but prized by patients still living in them forty years on. Predictably Abercrombie couldn't be afforded. What happened instead was widespread 'clearance' of the Victorian terraces and street patterns of Tower Hamlets, including many which were not damaged at all, and their replacement with 'comprehensive redevelopments'. But the good intentions of the local councils coupled with aspirations to Le Corbusier's principles and the social democratic building style of Sweden failed to produce much good architecture. The brick-built blocks characteristic of the philanthropic housing associations were regimented and grim but safe, soundproof and built to last. The classic LCC interwar estates although small in dimensions and quick to overcrowd with a tiny kitchen also had merits. When you visit them now, although tenants are cramped and the rooms are dark, they are warm and cosy. Indeed when they were built they must have stood out rather proudly from the low streets whose homes were unhygienic and lacked indoor sanitation, hot running water and privacy.

Certainly Morrison's achievement in rehousing a quarter of a million Londoners into 100,000 new homes at the height of the Depression shows what can be done. 'You got your own front door, a rent-book and a warm loo seat, it was Heaven,' a Stepney grandmother once told me, still remembering her delighted move into the Ocean Estate now in 1990 in terminal decay. An example of the long-promised planned rebuilding was the Lansbury Estate in Poplar, which was to house the contestants in the Commonwealth Games before it was handed over to the East End for housing. It has not matured well and was poorly and cheaply constructed with its visible metal and exposed concrete developing dampness, erosion and acoustic problems. But the overall plan did aim at a co-ordinated pattern of courtyards, green space and mixed scale of housing with social amenities planned into the original conception. If you had viewed Poplar, probably the area of maximum bomb damage, from one of the taller blocks on the Lansbury Estate by the late 1950s, despite arbitrary patches of overgrown bomb site and remaining sections of undemolished terraces, there would have been a sense of something new emerging from the devastation. There was an air of social optimism. And it was an urban community where people work, are educated, exercise and enjoy themselves, as well as are housed.

But Lansbury was unique and, largely for reasons of cost, this attempt at integrated planning was superseded by the tower block era's series of vertical 'units' which aimed to do little more than store people in concrete filing cabinets and then to wonder why they behaved antisocially when they got out. Industrialised building methods, now revealing extensive engineering defects, were used to spawn the tower block all over the inner East End and pepper Newham with the slabs. There is no doubt their building was systematically encouraged by central government subsidy and vigorous promotion by their Swedish originators. They also generated impressive statistics for the 'Never Had It So Good' Macmillan government, although many, including East End GPs like David Rosewarne, warned publicly of their antisocial effects. In Paul Harrison's curt synopsis: 'The idea: stand the street on its end so as to liberate the open space and greenery the city needs. The reality: malfunctioning lifts, vertigo, mothers terrified for children.' Nowadays such 1950s and 1960s blocks are typically approached, not via the welcoming parks of the artist's impressions, but through a semi-derelict and unfriendly open space with the odd incinerated litter bin, propped-up car and bashed-up swing to a grim entry porch, often impressively vandalised, with doors adrift and glass shattered.

In fact, once welcomed in on the fourteenth floor, the flat can be delightful. But while it might be desirable for young people who can cope with the access problems, it's a thoroughly hopeless place in which to bring up young children. When the lift goes, which is often, you have to use the emergency stairs. 'And what do you do,' a patient asked me, 'when, halfway up with shopping and a child and buggy, you realise you have forgotten the milk?' The sense of neighbourhood, of overlapping families and the close proximity of work, pub and play characteristic of the old East End courts and terraces, is turned into its opposite, a resentful proximity. The old terraces may have been unhygienic but they provided endless locations for social intercourse, gossip, courtship and news-gathering. It was a world whose scale made sense, where children might grow to know their nannies over the road and the character at no. 36 and which bar of which pub their uncle frequented. Instead the tower blocks froze people into well-upholstered isolation where the milkman won't deliver and the teenagers' first kisses are on the fire stairs. Once erected it seems to have been assumed that they would maintain themselves without the minimum of an on-site caretaker or concierge. So nothing seems to get done about the inevitable wear and tear any building is bound to sustain. Instead the stigmata of neglect remain; unrepaired mechanical breakdowns, dirty common areas, broken glass and tiles, ubiquitous foul graffiti. Then the belated improvements are mistreated and even the entryphones, meant as protection, are themselves vandalised. A building neglected by its landlord is unlikely to be respected by its tenants.

The social isolation in the tower blocks is offset by the famous East End markets – Crisp Street, the Roman, Petticoat Lane, Bethnal Green Road, Ridley Road, the Wastes in Hackney and Whitechapel – which retain the overcrowded intensity of prewar East London Life. As Ian Nairn put it in 1966: 'Of all the things done to London this century, the soft-spoken, this-is-good-for-you castration of the East End is the saddest. All the raucous, homely places go and are replaced by well-designed estates which would fit a New Town but are hopelessly out of place here. This is a hive of individualists, and the last place to be subjected to this kind of large-scale plan.' These antisocial features are even more prominent in the low-rise, high-density estates which succeeded the tower blocks. Typically their pattern is of interdigitating split-level maisonettes, approached by internal corridors without natural light. These corridors become infernal with regularly smashed light fittings, scorched, gouged and sometimes stripped-out linoleum, heavily embossed wall surfaces and stale smells. This handiwork is usually executed by passers-through who utilise the corridors and stairwells as meeting spots, skateboard or mountain bike runs, or glue- and heroin-sniffing stations.

While the conventional street gives the residents the psychological advantage of overlooking passers-by whose route and purpose are defined, the internal corridors give the initiative to the outsider. People soon get fed up of opening their (internal) front door in order to identify the noise-maker and instead live in a state of siege trying to ignore the public procession through the middle of their homes. Attempting to do home visits on this sort of estate, one often bangs and bells away for minutes until the heavily locked and shackled door is unbolted. Some residents illegally seal off access doors which makes the maze-like internal structure and numbering system even more incomprehensible, while still affording the knowledgeable assailant secure getaway routes. Visiting at night is both exasperating and frightening down these eerie, artificially lit, illogical corridors whose no. 6 can be two floors away from no. 7. And there is no worse mood in which to objectively examine and assess an ill patient. It is a relief, having successfully tracked down one's destination and extracted oneself from the consultation, to catch the night air and sudden

SOME LIVES!

complicated moon- and neon-lit vistas on the way back
to the car.

So what does the 'new East End' look like now from
the top of a tower block? There is no longer much
evidence of manufacturing industry, the chimneys and
cooling towers no longer billow smoke, the factories
are closed down and the freight yards stilled. On the
river there are a few odd pleasure and tourist boats and
an occasional empty water bus but the docks are dead
and the river, at least as a commercial and employing
force, is dying. The *Financial Times* printworks beams
an odd mixed light of pink and chrome across the A13,
casting soft shadows across the site of the old dockers'
Poplar Hospital in Brunswick Road, now long demolished. And the high-tech brick crates on the Isle of
Dogs which print the *Guardian* and the *Telegraph* now
they have moved out of Fleet Street throb in unison at
night. But the vast processing factories which used to
receive the Commonwealth trade along the river are
empty wrecks, their organ-pipe shafts decrepit and their
mock-Egyptian façades crumbling. Instead the container lorries pound and thunder down the Blackwall
Tunnel Approach creating a dull hum which can be
heard along a quarter-mile corridor either side on their
way to the Channel ports and up to the north of England. The electricity-generating station on Bow Creek
is closed and the Mill Meads gasworks run down. The
view eastwards is of car dumps, slaughterhouses, cemeteries and tower blocks. The odd new industrial estates
optimistically clad in brightly coloured, corrugated
plastic sited within inner East London are also largely
empty with forlorn 'To Let' signs offering acres of
industrial floorspace no-one can afford to utilise. With
supreme irony, the old Bryant & May factory, the site
of the matchgirls' strikes of 1889 which did so much
to spread the ideas of trade unionism to the unskilled
nineteenth-century East Enders, is being refurbished as
'Bow Quarter', a 'Manhattan-style' middle-class zone
of residential apartments.

Above it all twinkles the vast pointed obelisk of M. I. Pei's central block in the Canary Wharf complex, no. 1, Canada Square with its gleaming steel skin and green and red marble from Guatemala and Italy. It stands over East London like an uninvited guest at a party which is over. At its imperious ankles, new concrete motorways ramp and curl, Irish hard-hats, great-grand-sons of the men who built the docks, clamber, prowl and curse, and the light railway threads through a jumble sale of brightly coloured bits of box-and-crate architecture. To its feet come lorries, helicopters and barges laden with the enormous pre-built structures of modern construction and from it traffic jams steadily eddy outwards. But for all the investment and activity even Canary Wharf remains curiously alien, an attempt to parachute into the heart of the once industrial East End an identikit North American financial district. To outflank the City of London to its east was implausible enough at the height of the deregulation boom of the mid-1980s. To do so in an era of major recession with the property market collapsing round the Stock Market's ears seems impossible. But yet it hovers there, looking at night both beautiful and sinister, a gigantic Unidentified Fiscal Object, come to land on the old West India Dock.

Clearly the upriver docks had to change in character and probably contract. But there is much to be said in favour of working access by water to the heart of a capital city, especially one like London whose road network is being crushed by sheer weight of traffic (up 12 per cent between 1976 and 1988 despite a large fall in population). And land freed in such a central and historically important part of London clearly needed to be put to mixed uses including manufacturing and housing of a sort which would be of service to its existing population. But for the PLA the considerations appear to have been purely economic. The very rapid run-down of the Port of London in the 1960s, blamed on unofficial trade unionism, was a deliberate strategy to realise the rapidly rising value of the old dock area as a central commercial site ripe for redevelopment. And, in the course of the transfer to Tilbury, to decimate the labour force, shed office staff and neuter trade unionism. Although the dockers understood what was going on and attempted to put their case to the general public in the East End in a series of well-attended meetings, the PLA held all the cards. The redundancy terms seemed generous and the offer of jobs in Tilbury for those who wanted to stay on sounded solid: against union advice, most men went along with it. But the summary execution in barely two decades of the dock system which had sustained the waterfront boroughs for three centuries devastated not just the port but the associated industries and their communities. The great McDougall grain silo on the Millwall Dock which had pioneered the bulk hydraulic handling of flour had sustained many hundreds of jobs in Cubitt Town alone; it was one of the first to go, ceasing operation in the late 1940s. Tate & Lyle, the monopoly sugar refinery whose company town at Silvertown had employed 30,000 in 1955, finally shut down the Plaistow Wharf refinery in 1967. No more would East Enders flock to the famous Saturday Night Social Club or read Mr Cube's anti-nationalisation one-liners on the back of their breakfast sugar packet. The ship repair yards like Green and Silley Weir and Badgers closed in the mid-1970s. And the riverside food-processing, confectionery and biscuit manufacturers followed suit. Even the great brewing houses of the East End some five centuries old took the hint and upped and went. In the mid-1970s I was taken on a tour of the Manchester Road by women shop stewards campaigning against the closure of Poplar Hospital and we still addressed an audience of industrial workers, making speeches in ship repair canteens and car parks at the back of the gasworks, arguing with Sikh pattern-checkers and Irish pinewood-loaders. Of course, we couldn't win. One by one the hospital's facilities froze up, the consultants were bribed away

42

with the usual promises of better facilities in nearby hospitals. Poplar became a shell, expensively patrolled by guard dogs. But by the time it was finally demolished, all those industrial workplaces which had supported the campaign had gone too.

At first the scale of the job losses was disguised by an overall fall in the population due to a lower birth rate and the postwar out-migration to the New Towns and to Essex. In the textile industries and the furniture trades, although mass production methods devastated the smaller-scale artisanal East End workshops, the trades were able to keep going largely through a modern version of the highly cost-effective system of 'sweating', developed in the late nineteenth century and based, then as now, on the exploitation of the labour of recent immigrants and the low overheads of mainly female homeworkers in whose overcrowded council flats one often sees a shift-operated industrial sewing machine. The sweating system, an earlier variant of 'enterprise culture', was a persistence of pre-industrial petty manufacture. Instead of industrialised manufacturing where intensive capital investment could produce economies in mass production, small subcontractors contrive to keep their costs competitive by poor premises, bad working conditions, non-unionism, low wages and under-age and family labour. This sort of small-scale, highly exploitative production is endemic to East London and goes back to the seventeenth-century backyard, 'out-work' occupations of mattress-stuffing, brush-making, fancy goods manufacture and silk-winding.

The importance of work of this type in East London with its 'casual' nature, seasonal ebbs and inevitably low levels of trade union organisation can be over-stressed. The Beckton gasworks employed over 10,000 and was a famous centre of organised trade unionism and the Tate & Lyle sugar refinery was the biggest not just in Britain but in the world. But there were few new factories built in East London in the 1930s for the electrical and plastics industries, which expanded instead in the north-west of London. So the postwar East End employment pattern was unusually specialised with the majority in the docks and river-related industries and the remainder fairly equally subdivided between the food and drink industries, furniture-making and the rag trade.

So when the big job decline first hit London (in the decade 1961–1971, 31 per cent of manufacturing jobs were lost), Tower Hamlets was especially vulnerable with unemployment surging from a male level of 2.6 per cent and a female level of 1 per cent in 1961 to a male level of 6.2 per cent and a female level of 3.4 per cent in 1971. That rate of growth in unemployment accelerated during the recession of the early 1980s which drove out the few remaining major manufacturers that survived. And these high levels continued to grow remorselessly since the expansion in the late 1980s of the financial, property and retail sectors and the work brought to the East End by the LDDC had virtually nothing to offer local unskilled and semi-skilled workers and itself suffered in the recession of the 1990s. In fact the LDDC's net effect is probably to squeeze out more jobs than it has created, producing by the end of the 1980s formal male unemployment levels of 14.9 per cent whose true extent is probably between 20 and 25 per cent but among, say, Asian school-leavers is commonly over 40 per cent. Among one's patients, especially the over-fifties and the chronically sick, unemployment is a way of life and I have, with time, had to alter the question 'What is your job' to 'When did you last work?' Patients in work have to travel long distances, often to South and West London, even to work in supermarkets, offices and shoe shops. They are rarely members of trade unions, let alone active in them, and their employers, as well as paying them poorly, often demand private sick notes and penalise pregnant and ill patients with impunity. There is competition for previously low-status jobs like cleaning, the Post Office and road-sweeping. The council, the NHS itself and London Transport are now the major local employers; the banks, insurance companies and financial headquarters in the East End are mainly staffed from outside by clerks who commute, often by private coaches, from as far as Southend. The apprentice schemes which used to be so important in the East End, even if it was just to be a PLA messenger boy or a hairdresser, seem to have been largely wiped out, replaced by 'schemes' of negligible educational or skill content and short duration.

It's not sudden lack of ability or initiatives, in happier periods there have been plenty of East Enders who have made it, somehow, through the education system and are heads of advertising agencies, computer wizards, or professors of medicine. But the academic results achieved in East End schools were always low and are destined to get worse with the abolition of the ILEA, which skill-subsidised the poorer boroughs, and local management of schools, which requires managerial and academic experience uncommon among local parents. Skilled manual workers, often reluctantly, find they have to move out of the East End to live reasonably close to their work and many continue to emigrate (their mothers proudly show you snaps of them waving from the barbecues of Melbourne and the theme parks of California back at an incomprehensible England). So school-leavers who land jobs in the small local factories and warehouses which still function are unskilled machinists rather than fitters, forklift drivers rather than stores managers, till operators and shelf-fillers but never personnel managers. There's room but it's at the bottom. Because of the proximity of the City and the West End the employment picture is not quite as depressing as it might be for a similar port-based economy in the north-east or north-west. The black economy thrives and unofficial but lucrative dodging and diving continues. A bleak-looking minicab firm might well be operating all sorts of sidelines, the ill-lit leather workshop off Brick Lane may be supplying North Soho, the dustman, off duty, sells socks and shirts in the York Hall Turkish baths. And I still have patients happily working in the oldest of professions: actors, stonemasons, prostitutes and nurses. And despite all the dreadful documentary films about the contemporary East End with their lingering shots of waste paper wafting down broken pavements and bowed-down pensioners in bus queues, if you lift your head you can be startled by the beauty of the urban landscape in its diversity, vivacity and vast splendid skyscapes.

Cockney individualism, far from vanishing, as Ian Nairn feared, has become still more diverse if sometimes less obvious with the wild adaptations made by a multicultural proletariat and a sizeable bohemia. Once inside even the most forbidding tower block, East Enders still live in intricate little palaces with built-in bars, beautifully chosen hangings, curios and maxims and the gallery of family portraits. And sheer weight of concrete hasn't succeeded in abolishing East End conviviality: in the heat of the summer a family will sit, chatting, singing and drinking with their children on their front steps till past midnight. While opposite, their devout neighbours make prayers to Mecca.

Still, what always strikes me about those condescending documentaries about the poor East Enders, ignorant, ill and probably racist into the bargain, is exactly the reverse: how well the modern Cockneys do in circumstances which their 'betters' would find impossible. How much better they would do if their material conditions were hoisted a few notches up the class system. And yet how much more common decency, respect for humanity, honour and humour they possess than so many of the middle and upper classes who despite lip service to collective values in fact approach life in a spirit of naked self-interest. For this reason I agree with the doctor-poet William Carlos Williams who was a general practitioner in Paterson, an immigrant working-class town in New Jersey: 'I never felt that medicine interfered with me but rather it was my food and drink.'

CHAPTER 4

∞•◎•∞

A STAR IN THE EAST

Today a child was named after me. Bad enough if derived from a statesman or pop star. But a doctor should never need to be remembered in that way, just as pregnancy shouldn't be an illness. But this one is special, to me as well as its parents, one of twins, two boys, born by the test-tube baby technique to a thirty-nine-year-old mother who has wanted a family all her life. I knew the father first, a tall, distinguished-looking printer with a stiff walk, whose rebelliousness and early brushes with the law still stamp him with an independence of outlook and pride. He copes with a neck injury and asthma almost without complaint and stoically abandoned his beloved Norton for a beat-up transit van. I imagine he met his wife on motorbikes; they both have vintage biker tattoos and live together in one of the wartime flats which somehow never got rebuilt. Without any fuss, they love each other deeply. In winter their flat's freezing. And for a long time it's been missing a child.

Jeanette left having children till later than most East End girls; she was intelligent and had things of her own to do. And after she started trying for children, it took a long time for her to realise that she was infertile. No one was entirely sure why at first. It could have been an old fracture from a traffic accident she was lucky to survive as a girl, or a pelvic inflammatory disease from an unrecognised infection. But X-ray 'tie and die' examination on her Fallopian tubes finally showed that they were blocked on both sides. The only hope, it dawned on them, because the doctors didn't spell it out, was for an egg to be gathered (for the ovaries were still functioning normally) and fertilised outside the body. A test tube isn't in fact used but a Petri dish under microscopic control. But to get that done, if you are a buxom tattooed housewife and ex-Hell's Angel living in E14, isn't all that easy. When they started to look for help, in Harley Street, the technique was still experimental and far too expensive to consider. The techniques required aren't especially complex, but the fertility-enhancing drugs which are used to stimulate ovarian activity are costly. And these costs mount if it takes several attempts. And even then, there are a lot of failures. It's a procedure which utilises a lot of medical specialities, who all need to provide high-quality work and be used to co-operating with one another: X-ray, biochemistry, endocrinology and gynaecology. So it is tailor-made for an NHS hospital where all the different disciplines are already under one roof. It was, however, hard to find an In Vitro Fertilisation (IVF) set-up which would accept referral and, at that time, East London had no service of its own. Heartbreakingly, the South London centre which had them on the waiting list for two years had to write and tell them that cuts required it to restrict its services to the local area. And the next centre took four months to reply and turned out to have closed its list because of laboratory dificulties. By this time Jeanette had passed thirty-five, the magic cut-off age for entry into IVF. However, by complete chance, when I was attending an evening obstetrics refresher course, advance details of a new IVF centre accepting London-wide referrals were mentioned. So another ingratiating letter went off asking that the maternal age be waived, and they were admitted to another waiting list.

By this time it would have been wise to give up hope. But they didn't, continuing with a quiet certainty. They reported on their first contact with the hospital unit when allegedly coming into surgery for sore throats and repeat prescriptions, joking about the grim basement in which the IVF unit was housed. It was easy to imagine: quiet desperation being defused with cheerful tea and careful non-committal formulas. We arranged the fertility drug injections on GP prescriptions rather than the hospital's, not to save money but to transfer it from one part of the NHS budget to, then, a slightly less squeezed part. And glances were exchanged over the third prescription, because this would be Jeanette's last chance. So underneath the humour they were bracing themselves for sadness. Still hopeful, with that self-willed momentum people develop in such medical circumstances, but inwardly prepared for mourning for the loss of something they had never possessed.

Then the banal miracle. Jeanette missed her period and an ultrasound picked up not just one but two embryonic sacs. She bled at ten and then fourteen weeks and seemed to be miscarrying. Pete was terribly tense: a black volcanic mountain. He accompanied his wife to every appointment and blew up at an X-ray technician who was curt to her. So he and I had a row about being rude to X-ray technicians. Having had, and lost, children of my own, I understood a bit. But only a bit. Despite all the complications, they insisted on community-based antenatal care and went on seeing their consultant and midwife at the Health Centre. Always together, with their obstetric records pored over by Pete who would, I suspect, go home and double-check the charts, measurements and blood test results. There was concern towards the end of the pregnancy that one of the twins was failing to grow. It's not uncommon. And the ultrasound measurements of biparietal diameter and crown to rump length were now less useful than the ratio of skull diameter to abdominal girth.

While they sat watching us with mounting horror,

the consultant carefully replotted the ratios on the graph and convinced us all that both babies were still of good size. And so they were when eventually, after a twenty-hour labour, they were successfully delivered by caesarean section. When I first saw the babies back at home, perfectly duplicated and already like their proud parents, I wanted to cry because words, even 'joy' and 'happiness', seemed so hopelessly inexpressive. Attending medically during pregnancy never ceases to perplex. It begins so ambiguously: a 'missed' period. But inexorably comes evidence of a foetus germinating, then quickening, the softening and enlarging of the body to bear a child which is to be given out 'in labour'. 'Delivered' through the biggest door that is ever opened in life. Such joy and physical creativity after the vomiting, piles and stretching pains of pregnancy, the dreadful force of labour and the blood and shit and waters of birth. To the final shock and delight of suckling the immaculate, slippery, vernix-coated living being: the proof that bodies aren't just wonderful ideas but they *work*. Desire, sexuality, fertility. Intercourse, conception, procreation. The random sequence made circular and closed.

For doctors the activity comes at the beginning of the pregnancy and the end, in the crescendo of parturition. Inevitably, birth is an abstraction as one takes early blood specimens and examines heart, lungs and pelvis trying to be objective about what will be a highly emotional experience. For, medically, it's such an unpredictable undertaking, from the application of advanced technology, as in IVF or fetoscopy, to an uncomplicated pregnancy and a spontaneous normal delivery. Pregnancy goes wrong in the early stages more often than is realised (one in four pregnancies are said to miscarry) and there is surprisingly little that can be done medically about 'inevitable abortion'. Part of the paradox for a male doctor is one's knowledge that one will never experience the most important biological act that humans are capable of. Another is that one also spends a great deal of time and energy helping people not to get pregnant and arranging for the termination of unwelcome pregnancy. The number of abortions carried out in England and Wales rose from 174,276 in 1987 to 183,798 in 1988, as shown by the latest abortion statistics from the Office of Population Censuses and Surveys. The abortion rate amongst residents of England and Wales rose from 14.10 to 15.29 per 1,000 women aged 15–44. Twenty-three abortions were carried out above twenty-four weeks, eighteen on grounds of foetal abnormality.

Liberalisation of abortion law, notably in post-Franco Spain, means that fewer foreign women are forced to come to London for safe operations. The fact that the abortion rate continues to rise, especially in East London where the rate per 1,000 aged 15–44 is 20.06, must to some degree reflect several adverse features of modern living and less availability of contraceptive services. A continuing lack of adequate educational programmes in schools (health and sex education is *not* an obligatory part of the national curriculum) and continuing 'scares' and anxieties about the oral contraceptive, all combine to deter women from effective prevention of unwanted pregnancies. Many of the East End 'late' terminations are for teenagers, sometimes rape or incest victims, who have concealed their pregnancies. And an Asian sixteen-year-old recently got to term and delivered without her mother knowing, who then threw her out when she found out.

Still, some women, and certainly many husbands, choose not to limit families by the use of contraception. There is a long tradition of large families in the East End which probably relates to the preceding waves of immigration. Older white, often Irish-origin patients' family history frequently reveals families of eight or nine offspring, now geographically dispersed. And still-birth and the death of mother or child soon after delivery were also commonplace in East London until recently. The Tower Hamlets infant mortality rate (the

number of deaths of infants of less than one year old
per 1,000 total live births) which in the 1980s has ranged
between 10 and 16, is still significantly higher than
the England and Wales figures which average 11, and
appears to be increasing once again. Most European
countries have improved faster and more consistently.

This would confirm the long-held feeling that social
conditions, particularly the health and nutritional status
of the mother, rather than clinical innovation, are now
the determining factors in improving mortality. There
may be a residuum of congenital abnormality deaths
which will be improved only by better early detection
of foetal abnormalities by screening. But Tower Hamlets' high figures reflect the very steep gradation of
infant mortality according to social class: in England
and Wales the mortality rates in social class 5 are twice
those in social class 1. It is also connected to the number
of women having their first child in their teens and the
large families with short intervals between pregnancies.
These class gaps in mortality and family size are once
again widening. I kept a bedraggled notebook list of
the first twenty-three pregnancies I attended in E14
in 1985: only twelve proceeded to full-term normal
deliveries; there were five miscarriages, including two
late and very traumatic ones; four women chose to have
abortions; there was one stillbirth and one neonatal
death. Compared with the endless production of
healthy young babies at the Kent district hospital where
I had recently been training, it seemed, and was,
another world.

And in obstetric practice in East London it is rare
to see the sort of 'normal' family portrayed by the
manufacturers of nappies, soap powders and breakfast
cereals: white, married, with a small, well-planned
family. Instead, a typical antenatal clinic will have a
majority of mothers themselves born in Bangladesh,
Vietnam and North Africa. Many British-born white
and Afro-Caribbean mothers will be unmarried and
usually living in the overcrowded parental home.

Marriage is commonly postponed until the birth of the second or third child, if at all. For the teenagers, getting pregnant has often been a fairly passive experience: unprotected intercourse with a transitory boyfriend. But it is also, for a schoolgirl who isn't good at school, a startling change in status. She is, in one bound, a woman, suddenly the centre of attention and curiosity. All the complicated processes and crises of maturation are pushed out of the way, indefinitely postponed as the pregnancy presses on, stopping, once established, for no-one. How much time there will be to repent at leisure.

It's not the case that all young mothers do badly; they often show astonishing maturity. But the sugary side of being pregnant, the goo-goo ga-gas and knitted matinee coats, is overwhelmed by starker forces: the exhaustion, the weight, the sheer work of labour. And when birth is over, the business of watching a child grow and establishing a relation to it when you are emotionally and intellectually still emerging from childhood yourself, is immense. It is absurdly easy to conceive. But so prodigiously difficult to be a good parent. Especially when your parents are staring over your maternal shoulder all the time. One lass, Irene, reticent to the point of invisibility, pitched up four months gone, towed in by a furious mother. She mumbled that she didn't know how she had got pregnant and one almost believed her, such was her perennial vagueness. Irene was just the sort of girl who gets taken advantage of. She was absolutely emphatic that she wanted the child and unrepentantly forgetful about the boy's identity.

But as the pregnancy advanced, she seemed almost to lose herself inside it. After delivery, the hospital midwives thought, wrongly, that she was mentally subnormal and asked a psychiatrist to see her. In her little ill-lit bedroom, she had carefully assembled the paraphernalia of child care, a veritable chariot-borne trousseau of oils, tissues and perfume. Entering this room was like going into a little chapel: the crib the altar, the nappies sacraments, fragrant talc the incense. 'Is everything OK?' 'Yes, Doctor.' Then suddenly awash with tears. About breastfeeding. Guilty about failing. But unable to get an exhausted, hungry baby to fix properly. I should have sat down and shown her. Stayed with her till it went right. Waited for the avid baby and overwhelmed mother to get the feelings and the rhythms right. I should have been able to understand the great hurricane of feelings and of hormones that whirl about in the days after delivery. Instead I fussed about how overheated the bedroom was as the tears slopped down her face, once 'plain', now beautiful in her fecundity. The midwife had shared the hospital's concern and thought she should be readmitted to hospital, which she had hated. The damning phrase 'postnatal depression' was whispered. But to send her back to hospital would have been to confirm her in the incompetence which everyone was busy assuming for her. So we took swabs from everywhere, since a skin infection might have been causing the feeding difficulties, and visited the egg box twice daily, while slowly and surely the rash faded and the breastfeeding succeeded. And in a month there she was, beaming in the baby clinic, chattering to new friends and arranging a branch of the One O'Clock club.

Experience in obstetric matters is an unreliable teacher. Another mother of the same age, destined, the school thought, for a college place, brimmed with vivacity and intelligence. But she had managed to fall in love with a good-looking lout who pinched her pocket money for heroin and hit her when she protested. Undeterred, she declared herself homeless and took the 'reformed' boyfriend for the qualifying purgatory in a Hammersmith bed-and-breakfast. But couldn't stand cooking smells in the bedrooms and came back to the East End during the day, while he drifted back to heroin, thence to stealing, thence to violence and 'the police being called'. Her persona was so competent, despite the evidence that she consistently got herself into daft situations, that she never needed help, she thought. But was constantly attended for trivial physical problems to do with somatised anxiety, and often panicked during her pregnancy, once calling from a phone box imagining she was miscarrying, when she actually had a bleeding pile. Under the pressure, she had 'funny turns', went still like a statue and heard voices. When the baby was delivered, unable to endure the procedure of hostel boarding-out necessary to become officially homeless, she returned home and soldiered on with a child who became progressively insomniac, eczematous and plain hard to handle. And in turn became more unhappy as the implications of what had happened to her sunk in: her teenage years taken away from her, her ambitions curbed, her baby no longer the sweetly smiling dreamboat of the congratulations card, but a screaming, insatiable brat. But, like Irene, she retained a vitality which is particular to East End women, and could be spellbindingly quick and articulate about her own frustration. And I think of another mother, ex-heroin addict, dependent on opiate and benzodiazipine tablets, who, with her husband who had his arm amputated because of dirty shared needles, kicked completely when she became pregnant. There is such force in these encounters that one has to delve inside oneself to find ways of meeting it.

It's the first year, when everything has to be given in an unending donation, that demands so much and breaks so many parents' spirits. It is a long haul till the little beans finally get off to school and, apart from the endless giving, there's not a lot to look forward to. No wonder that sometimes the young mothers manage for the first two years and then suddenly up and go; hand over their child to the grandparents and walk out. For the 'preparation for pregnancy' isn't really about breathing patterns during labour or hints on how to wash the baby. It's about the immense transition that the business of becoming a parent, for which none of us is properly prepared, involves. It is like acquiring a new limb. But a limb which has a life of its own and, while objectively dependent, fights implacably for its independence.

It's also about the shock of parturition: the nagging discomfort of the early stages, the private world of painful dilation in the second, and the absolute delight of pushing out, unfettered and releasing at last. 'I can see the head' must be the most marvellous five words in the language after a pregnancy of three seasons and a labour of a day: you are finally there, at the grand finale after all that aching and waiting. And there is your slippery, bloody, airborne offspring. Birth is an elemental, terrifying, violently emotional release. You can't deodorise it: there's the squit of faeces as the head comes down, and the blood as the perineum tears, and the coat of vernix caseosa in which the baby is enveloped. It is about blood and sweat and tears as well as joy. It's also about risk and the proximity of death. The Workers' Birth Control Group used to campaign in the 1920s under the slogan that it was twenty times as dangerous to have a baby as to go down a mine. In modern Britain, delivery is now much safer, but this for East End mothers is a relatively recent historical development and still does not apply in large parts of the world. The words of Pozzo in *Waiting for Godot* are literal: 'They give birth astride of a grave, the light gleams for an instant, then it's night once more.'

The domestication of pregnancy is highlighted when a baby does die in hospital. Because a labour ward doesn't know how to deal with death: the producer of a dead baby is in the wrong place. It's then that people really do go to pieces. But wouldn't have to if we weren't all so keen on normality and thus on the tidying-away of extreme unintelligible experience. People used not to be even shown the dead baby. Instead something would be said about 'Nature's way of dealing with imperfection', and the mother would be sent home emptyhanded to contemplate her layette. And

fantasise about her baby: fantasies which would
invariably be worse than any reality. Now parents are
encouraged to be with their child when it dies, to hold
it and to name it. Polaroid pictures of skinny mites with
drips in incubators can now have their rightful place
among the family portraits round the mirror and parents can grieve rather than just amputate their feelings
and 'try again'. That doctors and midwives should have
ever had the impertinence to do otherwise is an index of
quite how depersonalised 'scientific' medicine became at
its postwar apogee.

The delight at a successful birth, however disguised
in mawkish congratulation, confectionery and upholstered cards, is a passionate congratulation on the
success of labour, on delivery, on the creation of new
life, the most important but most unrecognised activity
humans undertake. And a recognition of the dangers
that have been overcome. East Enders' apparent sentimentality over new babies is in fact their recognition
of what is truly important in life. There is therefore
nothing more delightful than a new birth visit, even if
it is obvious that the mother is already fed up with the
doorbell ringing with flowers or well-wishers. You are
always recognised and welcome because not a visitor
but a fellow traveller. In theory it's an important medical chance to recheck the baby's hips, heart and general
health. And to review the mother's mental and physical
state. But, that done, it is a time to share and congratu-
late. To look the baby in the eye and see it blinking at
the light. To count its minute wrinkled digits and
wonder how come there are always five. To look again
at palate, brow and palms to exclude, yet again, congenital disease. To squeeze the mother and clap the
father on the shoulders in salute of what they have
done. And to leave by the lift or the street mysteriously
elated but also quite relieved to be free of the cloying-
ness. Thus a new birth visit is a kind of acted ritual, a
mime of congratulation (because one knows what is
ahead) and a calculation (because what one is really

thinking about is the necessary banalities of contraception, scalp lotions and nappy rashes). But then you might next be visiting a patient, whom you also have come to know, who is dying.

The distinctions of class are sharp even at birth. The gulf is most marked in the private health systems. In California the rich can have all forms of exotic delivery, while the country as a whole is twentieth down on the list in child mortality, and babies die for want of proper antenatal facilities. But in Britain, most middle-class mothers have their baby on the NHS. Although the event is biologically similar, the experience is different. Middle-class mothers have their children much later, commonly in their thirties, and have smaller families. They treat doctor and midwife more questioningly, might have a birth plan (which almost invariably doesn't match the birth at all) and sit in antenatal clinics buried in a paperback birth book. In a way, the working-class 'take it as it comes' attitude is probably a more flexible philosophy with which to enter the immense uncertainty of delivery than a written-down birth plan. This is not a question of 'natural childbirth' versus hospital authoritarianism; still less of men versus women. Rather, it's the strange belief of the educated middle class that events can be somehow controlled by reading the literature and writing down one's preferences, as one might consult the *Good Food Guide* and then order what *you* want from the menu, ignoring the intimidating suggestions of the waiter. There is nothing sadder than a couple whose written plan, designed to avoid analgesia or obstetric intervention, crumples in failure to progress after a long labour on bean bag or birth stool and bent double. It was, after all, the progressives in the women's movement who fought for access to high-quality hospital care because of their experience of long, unproductive home deliveries, sickly neonates and exhausted, poorly nourished working-class mothers.

The middle-class new birth visit is also to a slightly

different world. Baby is still centre-stage and the delight
and pride are common. But baby will already be clad in
gender non-specific primary colours and its first toys
will be non-sweetening, design-award-winning,
psychologically appropriate mobiles rather than the
pink or blue cuddly toys which arrive in the crib of the
proletarian newborn. Class assigns self-confidence, but
there is no reason why a headmistress in N16 is going
to be more proficient as a mother than a seventeen-
year-old in E14. A degree doesn't make a baby's night-
time cry any the less piercing or soothe a stinging episi-
otomy. Middle-class men are by no means better fathers
or spouses than working-class men. In fact, they are
more likely to have to go back to work quickly and to
have jobs which leave them little sympathy with the
baby-zone of feelings. But class realities affect child care
rapidly. A little child's prodigious and promiscuous
needs isolate and infantilise anyone who deals with
them singlehandedly. The key to looking after children,
as the working-class extended family realised, is to have
as many adults and others involved in the task as possible. Getting out, even if it's just to the doctor for
the six-week check, is both physically and emotionally
tiring when the journey has to be made with a buggy
on a crowded bus or down cold dirty stairways. A car,
parents with a home outside the city, the telephone, a
husband who can come home early or go in late after
a bad night, make a big difference.

The reality of East End working-class life is quite
different. A husband who is working at a labouring job
for long hours and gets home exhausted. A mother
who will have a sewing machine or other out-work
sharing the baby's room with the cot. A large proportion of young single mothers trying to share an
already overcrowded council flat with their parents and
sisters, and only a tiny giro income of their own. It's a
world with little privacy, cramped space, no garden
retreat. Money is short and intermittent, so what's left
after the basics is spent improvidently on treats and

cheer-ups. So there may be a video, but not many toys and few books. There could be a shiny chrome and leather studio sofa from a sale and a nice carpet from a door-to-door dealer; but no tumbledryer or dishwasher and a washing machine which regularly packs up. Established Cockneys still, despite the housing, tenaciously hold together in extended family patterns and know how to help young parents: West Indians are particularly strong family visitors. And Cockney grandfathers take their responsibilities to their grandchildren seriously. But recent immigrants have grandparents or aunties who are back home. So, since permission to enter Britain on a family visit is so hard to obtain from Dacca, it is customary for young Bangladeshi children to make an extended visit with their parents to meet their family. It is because of the length of this trip that many Bangladeshis resident in Tower Hamlets have been evicted for making themselves 'intentionally homeless'.

The larger immigrant family home is still more likely to be overcrowded with children sharing beds, several to a bedroom, father working shifts and overtime to bring in an income, mother and elder girls homeworking rather than doing their homework, the family fed monotonous, overcooked, starched and fat-rich food from pans permanently on the stove. In the circumstances, what is remarkable is how clean and healthy the children are. Indeed, presumably because of the powerful aspirations of parents who have made this risky, frightening leap to live in London, one is often approached about children who are quite normal in weight and height for their years, with the fear that they are 'too small' or 'don't eat anything'.

'Infant welfare' has echoes of cod-liver oil and queuing for the needle or the lump of sugar. For medical students and doctors it has low status despite requiring a high level of clinical expertise and being a cost-effective means of improving public health and life expectancy. Perhaps this is because, like so much screening and preventive work, it depends on unglamorous routine with little chance for diagnostic coups. Breakthroughs do exist: there has been a dramatic increase in the survival rate for children suffering from kidney cancer and leukaemia. Overall death from cancer for children under fourteen years has fallen by a quarter since 1961. However, these cancers account for a small proportion of total children's deaths, with accidents and respiratory disease showing much larger and more sharply class-related patterns. And poor hygiene, inaccurate feeding knowledge, overcrowding, poor nutrition and parental smoking are much more likely to lead a child into a cycle of repeated minor illness.

The aim of infant welfare policies and child health clinics was originally to effect an overall improvement in the health of under-fives as the most effective way to improve the well-being of the whole population. It is what founders of the 1930s Peckham experiment in community health called 'the cultivation of the social soil in which the families were growing', looking at 'ethos' rather than 'pathos'. It was very much part of the postwar social optimism which pioneered the NHS, free school milk, the first custom-built comprehensive schools, health visitors, baby clinics and cod-liver oil. It is now somewhat ruined social territory, dive-bombed in the Thatcher years, unreconstructed by Major, waiting, with little enthusiasm, for Kinnock. The consequences of its destruction – less healthy, less stable and less educated children – are identified and dealt with by the state, of course. But ten years too late, by policemen, dole officers, prison warders and coroners' courts instead of teachers, school nurses and GPs.

Vaccinations are the most mundane part of preventive child health, but immunisation remains important and difficult in the East End. There are regular measles epidemics with, in some cases, severe complications which should have been prevented by effective vaccination. Measles is a preventable and unpleasant childhood illness which is a significant cause of death. Whooping cough, too, is not uncommon, with that exhausting, high-pitched bark of a cough which can continue for up to eight weeks. The children who catch it are largely those whose parents refused vaccination after the scare about possible brain damage in the late 1970s. The relatively low uptake of vaccine is due to health professionals giving inaccurate advice about the categories of people who ought to avoid the pertussis vaccine. Another challenge in vaccination is the dis- covery in antenatal screening that some East End mothers from Vietnam have suffered in the past from a type of hepatitis which can cause long-term liver cancer. Although not very contagious, it can be passed from mother to child. So any child born to a mother who is Hep. B positive needs to have a course of six immunisations in the first year to become immune. Tuberculosis, an infectious illness closely associated with poor living standards, is still commonly diagnosed in the East End, although eliminated in most of Britain. So children who might visit India or Bangladesh, Hong Kong or the Caribbean, or who have a family history of TB, are also vaccinated at six weeks.

An injection clinic, like all medical procedures, can be done well or badly. But it's not very pleasant to spend a morning inflicting pain on trusting little inno- cents who can't understand why on earth you are being so cruel, even if their parents do. It's optimistic that so many non-English-speaking mothers bring their children up to these clinics with so little tangible to gain. Presumably they have firsthand experience of infant mortality from infectious illness in their countries of origin and appreciate the value of vaccination. At the end of 1988, Tower Hamlets was one of twenty-five health districts in Britain publicly listed by the Depart- ment of Health as having the worst rate of vaccination in Britain. This probably reflects many factors of unequal weight including poor social conditions, out- of-date information on the part of both parents and health workers, language problems, patchy child health clinics, high mobility, backward GP services and sheer weight of numbers. It is quite obviously a more demanding procedure to get a genuinely informed consent for a triple vaccination from a non-English-speaking Vietnamese mother of four, who has had to walk with all her kids to surgery and wait an hour, than in the leafy suburbs.

Still more demanding is the accurate assessment of developmental milestones in small children which lies at the heart of successful community paediatrics. The clinical signs – heart murmurs, bow legs, hip instability, muscular tension, or failure to gain appropriate weight – can be elicited, with some difficulty, without the means of verbal communication. Though even here it is necessary to adjust weight parameters to take into account the smaller heights of Asian parents. But since a lot of paediatric assessment depends on parental obser-vation, communication problems abound. If there is no independent translator, both parent and doctor can overcompensate by imagining communication or with-draw into a passive, incomprehending gloom. At the six-week check, it is desirable to distinguish between the general smile a newborn child will confer indis-criminately upon the world, and the smile of recog-nition it will produce for its mother as an early learned reflex. Which is quite a complex distinction to explain.

From its first lung-clearing squall, the child has been grappling productively with the outside world. In its first six weeks, underneath the silly adult ceremonies and matinee coats, the newborn's neurology is surging, exploring, responding, learning. Its visual field, flooded with the light-show of life, is winnowing systematically through that bombardment, finding focus and the beginning of perspective, identifying the eternal curves of faces, lips and breast, starting the lifelong process of colour association. Its back and neck begin to brace themselves against gravity and in relation to position, to develop the reflexes and tone which are, unrealised by adults, constantly measuring and calculating to make possible posture. Its lungs are finding out how to suck and cough and cry. It is hearing the pandemonium of the noisy world outside the echo chamber of the pregnant abdomen and, instead of fearing it, begins to imitate it. It experiences cold and wet and soft and warm. It gulps and sucks and shits and pees, with its hands, those most fascinating pieces of neurology, grappling, like the irons thrown over the sides of ships of war, with the grip of grim death, holding on to whatever comes within what is now its grasp.

So by the great age of the six-week check, the child has already graduated in its own university of the senses and so far developed from the newborn to be clinically unrecognisable. To watch a doctor perform a six-week check you might think nothing of it. Baby hoisted and twirled a few times, hips cocked and braced open, a light shone, the stethoscope brandished, a groin palpated and that's it. But by demonstrating the loss of some of the primitive reflexes present at birth and their replacement by new responses, one is authenticating the first rites of neurological passage. And when the naked baby is lifted across the room in the examiner's hand 'in ventral suspension', alarmingly as if to be launched into flight like a paper dart, the ability of the head to ascend level with the plane of the body is the evidence of six weeks' hard labouring to learn head control. So obtaining the 'red reflex' excludes cataract, demonstrating the ability to 'fix', that is, engage the examining doctor's eye, and detecting the quick flicker of the femoral pulse are clinical signs of great import. And already at six weeks, the fearless symmetry of the responsive child who smiles and stills to its mother's voice is that of a little grown-up.

And by ten months, the time of the next formal development check, much has happened. Biting, chewing, holding. Rattling, poking and inspection. The baby now sits, omnipotent, surveying its conceptual kingdom, its babble now bi-syllabled and on the way to speech. It is now persistently hauling itself to the standing position. Not only have its length, weight and head circumference clambered up the curves of the centile chart but it's now making its first forays into emotional responses, feelings more complex than the megalomaniac expression of its own lacks, needs and pleasures. It has begun the lifelong work of understanding the differences in the emotional tones of the human voice, that most superbly expressive of instruments. And learning how to live with others, that other lifelong work.

Mostly the kids make their own way up to the miniaturised adults which are normal five-year-olds. There is wide variation with similar eventual outcomes (the late walking child might be the bright one, working harder on its brain than its leg muscles). One only realises the immense intellectual and physical work that is 'normal' development when a defector is unmasked: the emotionally deprived child who fails to gain weight and falls away from the orderly curves of the weight charts, the motor-delayed whose tone is floppy and who can't stay sat upright at ten months, the spastic whose limbs become stiffened and cock-eyed and who squints and slurps its speech. And requires the painful recognition by its parents that things are going to be a very different ascent. That perhaps spoonfeeding will still be needed at twelve, that clear speech will never be shared although a private language might be gained, and that the beautiful child will live inside a body that jerks and jiggles all its life. In fact, a linear sequence of skill attainment implicit in the classical development tests, with their tasks of piling bricks and identifying objects, is an illogical way of monitoring the emergence of functional co-ordination. Rather, child development occurs in a pattern of refractory stages and breakthroughs which relate interactively with the outside world. And the family in turn recentres itself in relation to its latest member. It's easy to watch skin filling out to replace the wrinkles of the newborn, to notice meaningful smiles of recognition, annotate the first babytalk and observe that most fascinating of reflexes, the human grip, grow in assurance and precision. Indeed, there is something infinitely satisfying in plotting a steady curve of weight increase against national centiles. Or watching the baby who could only suck or cast away an offered brick, imitate and then pile them. But that doesn't tell you enough about what is going on in that family's life. Children are born perfect-bodied but without any power of mental discrimination. Not the *tabula rasa*, the open book of Roman belief exactly, but an omnivorous, highly alert brain for which all is grist to the sensory mill. The age at which a child takes its first step is easy to record but doesn't relate at all to its eventual intelligence, happiness, or even athletic skill. An unhappy or ill-treated child will tend to lose weight which it will promptly regain if looked after properly and with affection, even if that is by a stranger. But it is possible to see quite soon whether a child is going to reach its full human potential. And the answer in East London is invariably no.

This is not the fault of the parents. In one sense a child is born as old as its parents: it has access to all of their experience, their wisdom and their capacity for love. So if your parents are too young, or preoccupied with making ends meet, or overwhelmed with the demands of other children, that can't be altered with a pill or a jab. And if they have been damaged emotionally or are depressed, it will be hard for them to love and to calm you. But then parental maturity, patience and ability to concentrate, listen and encourage, in turn depend on a series of material factors: the quality of their education, their security in childhood, their housing conditions, their status at work, type of job and income. It is expecting rather a lot of a young mother who left school to have her baby, suddenly, by virtue of procreation, to equip herself with tolerance, patience and a capacity for reciprocity no-one else in the world possesses. To cope at all is remarkable.

So the very marked differences in deaths of under-fives according to social class make sense as social geography rather than individual skill or ability. If you live on an inner city council estate, although unlikely to be a car owner, you will live in an area of heavy traffic. While having an overcrowded flat, there will, typically, be little safe supervised playspace such as a private garden provides. What playgrounds there are will often be distinctly unsafe, with equipment in poor repair and with derelicts and homeless people in residence. So children, from a very early age, are shouted at and hit indoors because they inevitably get in the adults' way or in places of danger. They are more likely to be thrown on their own devices or grudgingly be supervised by elder brother or sister during holidays and after school. And there is a greater likelihood of an accidental domestic fire due to cheap or out-of-date electrical equipment and flammable furniture. As the Black Report puts it: 'It is impossible to escape the conclusion that in the context of childhood the most straightforward of material explanations is capable of providing a simple chain of causation by which the pattern of health inequality is illuminated.'

Class is stamped even at the breast and in the buggy. As in late Victorian England, in the late twentieth century the well-off have greatly elaborated and refined their domestic food as well as restaurant facilities. Although it might be the microwave rather than a maid, there is a world of difference between their fresh, well-cooked and nutritious intake and the supermarket trolleys of the obese poor, full of cheap sweeteners and quick fillers. The contrast between the diet of the social classes is not, as perhaps it once was, a matter of quantity. Rather, the well-off spend more on a smaller quantity and eat out, with their children, more often. Large poor families have relatively little fresh fruit available, and salads, fish and poultry are rare. Instead, processed meats, served as reheated sausages and pies, lard, sugar and jam are prominent and convenience food is universal. 'Eating out' means a hamburger or a pizza during a shopping expedition. The sheer time and organisation required to cook complex recipes are not present and children, being quick learners and gastronomic conservatives, tend to demand what they know.

Immigrant families, even those who come from areas where obesity is uncommon and food scarcity has devolved a cuisine of which the nutritionalists approve (like China where protein is sparingly combined with lightly cooked vegetables and rice), acquire the worst of Western habits fast. Schoolkids' eating habits merge, with more than three-quarters of 10–15-year-olds having fat intakes above the recommended level of 35 per cent, more than half of that obtained from chips, crisps, biscuits, chocolate and burgers. Clearly the combined effect of intensive advertising and the abolition of standard nutritional specifications for school meals in 1980 have exerted a malign effect.

At a time when leisure shopping has become a new sort of entertainment for the credit-card classes, low pay, shrinking welfare benefits and high unemployment make the supermarket visit a matter of quick stomach-filling for the urban poor. In the East End this is manifest in the stark contrast between the home-delivered champagne and gourmet services in the brochures of the LDDC and the arrays of pop, oven-ready chips and burgers in the general store, or in the opulence of Tobacco Wharf with its malls of status objects and the grimness of the East End corner shops and dismal rows of off licence, video shop, tobacconist and minimart. The final twist is that the prices charged in the corner store or mobile shop with its small unhealthy range are in fact higher per item than in the suburban shopping malls. In promotion, the contest is unequal. In 1985, Rowntree Mackintosh, Mars and Cadbury together spent £66.7 million on advertisements, while the entire Health Education Council's budget for promotion of healthy eating in the same year was only £750,000.

As with food, so with toys and books and outings.

In a way the quantity of the toys or their cost make little difference if children aren't helped and encouraged to play with them. A box of poster paints and a brush, providing there is an adult who has the time and space to help, is a most luxurious toy. But East End homes tend to have a lot of cheap toys, often heavily TV-promoted, which quickly break or lose their novelty value. Around Christmas the waste bins overflow with wrapping paper and cartons, but toys given with the impetuous generosity which is one of the East End's most endearing characteristics, are out of commission by New Year. And the desperation to keep a crowded house clean rules out the most useful play for young children, that which requires mess, spillage and mud. And leads to the endless East End litany of threat and then punishment to which the children have become habituated and which they learn to ignore and endure: 'If you don't stop doing that at once I'll wallop you!' or 'If you don't stop doing that, the doctor will stick a needle into you.' Wallop.

Children's bedrooms, because they are multi-occupied, are seldom equipped for individual play or homework, which tend to take place in front of a TV which is permanently switched on, in front of which dogs scratch and adults smoke, drink and argue. In small doses it's cheerfully communal. As a way of life, it's very hard on children who, apparently treated as honorary adults, are in fact denied their own separate sphere and recognition. Teenagers particularly hate it and brave cold corridors, lift shafts and car parks just to get out of the oppressively static fug. And children grow up together, whether they like it or not. East London has no place for a shy or solitary child; cohabitation is compulsory. In the process they learn unpleasant things from each other: that the neighbourhood is rough and disliked by those who live in it, that all the children go short, that parents are unpredictable and often rough, that love is provisional and unreliable, that bullies get away with it and that pain makes you cry.

70

A common pattern is for children to be allowed to stay up late to watch TV they don't understand, largely because no-one can make the effort to put them to bed. The family then lie in, missing school, and bleary-eyed in night clothes start another day of TV, cigarettes and lager with the midday news. The absence of children's books is marked, despite the attempts of schools to encourage library borrowing, reading schemes and book purchase saving clubs. In the whole of Tower Hamlets, population 166,000, I know of only two bookshops, inconveniently situated in the north-west of the borough, although several newsagents and super-markets have pulp paperback sections. The culture of the book and the habit of reading, so important to Jewish self-improvement in the East End, are in retreat before the comic, the magazine and the video. Children of all national origins recognise children's book charac-ters only if they have appeared in a TV or cartoon format: so Superted but not Noddy. Of course, there is something alarming about the book-pushing of some middle-class parents which seems to want to turn children into precocious miniature adults. Sometimes it's as if the middle classes treat their children as their puppets and the working class talk to their children as if they are lovable but disobedient pets. Which is worse?

As for holidays, a significant number of families simply can't afford to take them. Better-off East Enders have a long tradition of buying caravans in the Essex estuary where they can garden and watch TV with fresher air and a view of the oil depots of Canvey Island. But often, when an East End mother is asked when she last had a proper holiday, she looks blank and then remembers staying with relatives a year or two ago. One of the results of the postwar working-class improvement in living standards was the confidence it gave people to explore and utilise the countryside and overcome the habits of metropolitan parochialism. Through Outward Bound, scouting and the Municipal Adventure Course, mountaineering, exploring, canoe-

ing and fen walking ceased to be largely the preserve
of the middle classes. This was part of a process which
goes back to the bicycle, that symbol of emancipation,
and derives from the working-class sport and rambling
associations of the interwar period. And East Londoners
had always had their own country holidays: the hop
weeks when special trains took families for an outdoor
fortnight of open air work, camp fire and unsupervised
sleeping arrangements. But hopping was industrialised;
the holiday business became increasingly commercial-
ised, and by the 1960s the typical East End holiday was
the package to Torremolinos or Ibiza. And even on the
British holiday beaches a not very subtle segregation
operated: Southwold and Aldeburgh, unspoiled and
slightly inaccessible, for the birdwatching and music-
loving middle classes; Southend and Clacton for candy-
floss, amusements and a beach as crowded as the Roman
Road. For getting away from it all on a package doesn't
get very far if the food is English, the hotels are like
tower blocks and the beaches are polluted and packed.
If you see a school trip of inner city schoolkids on the
beach at Frinton, it is as foreign to them as Red Square
or the Eiffel Tower. And, sadly, they as foreign to it.

CHAPTER 5

GROWING UP TOUGH

So an East End child's life is still tough. In microcosm it can be seen every weekend in a pub's children's room. Here mum, prematurely old in the face, already overweight and slack in dress and carpet slippers, sits head in hands, opposite dad who's already into his fourth pint, and blows cigarette smoke reflectively into it. Her three children are ignored and out of mind: one desperately attention-seeks and punches and kicks his fellows on the climbing frame while his sister quietly sobs to herself in the queue for the video game. Or see the depressed mother the next day slumped in the surgery waiting room, impervious to her amok offspring.

None of this is to disparage proletarian family life. It has a generosity and emotional directness strikingly absent from the conventional middle-class family. The proletarian home, because it is inherently uncomfortable and has to fight for its existence at every turn, is both more passionate and more sensible, with a set of values which correspond to real social worth. The home of the immigrant worker is marked by a determination and an immense struggle for identity which is both painful and beautiful to watch. And in the East End, because of the long history of men working in short-term and in seasonal employment, women are more assertive, responsible and self-confident. This may lead to conflict but is healthier, for parents and children, than the ingrained belief in the inferiority of the woman present in Scotland and some parts of the industrial north.

But it would be ill-advised to be sentimental about these good traits since they are so easily undermined by material circumstances and mutate into something less appealing. The communalism can easily become an oppressive lack of privacy. The daily struggle for survival, permanently pitted against the next problem, becomes exhausting after years; demoralising and embittering when carried on decade after decade. The generous spirit and sense of decency which distinguish even the poorest of the working class are seldom explicitly socialist views but are their prerequisite. In many ways the problem is that people simply don't have the institutions and the time with which to assemble a political point of view. But there is a palpable set of East End values: that you shouldn't jump the queue, that you are not just in it for yourself, that it's right to help people in trouble and that loyalties matter more than cash. Together they mean a solidarity, if not of factory or union branch, then of everyday life. Often they are expressed most strongly where children are concerned. But these beliefs are under attack every day by a highly coherent commercial culture which has a price for everything but knows nothing's value. They inevitably break down into a muddle of incentives and optings-out and couldn't-care-lesses. It rains demands and the streets are awash with despair. So why not do as the culture says? Do your own thing rather than do the right thing. And then wonder why you can no longer assemble anything from the bits and pieces of identity you can salvage. And discover you have nothing to give to your children that works without batteries.

It is possible to measure the incidence of ill-health in East London to demonstrate that before they are five, twice as many will have died of accidents and fires, cancers and chest infections as the children in Bromley five miles down the Blackwall Tunnel. It is possible to deduce some reasons why. Some are simple: about traffic density and overcrowding and lack of safe, supervised playspace, about housing policy and leisure facilities. Which is, in turn, about class. Something very simple but apparently very hard to alter in a society which has inverted the social optimism of the postwar years into a complete pessimism and uninterest in anything that isn't done by individual effort. Some answers are more complicated than simple impoverishment: they are about cumulative patterns of deprivation, about cycles of ill-health. East End babies have more respiratory problems, in part because heavy cigarette smoking is persisting longer here than in middle-class London. But that in turn needs explanation. It is much harder to give up a cheap, heavily advertised, addictive, stress-relieving drug if you also live in indifferent housing, have a low income, have very little respite from stress and completely lack time to take stock and work out new directions. Anyway, respiratory problems persist even when you do manage to give up because they are also due to atmospheric pollution, damp housing, inherited lung disease due to parental occupation and other things willpower can't shake. Both the rich and the poor indulge in harmful habits; the poor just possess fewer alternative rewards and feel they have a lot less to lose. Some of these inequalities, especially the carcinomas, may obey geographical rather than sociological laws and relate to toxins and industrial and nuclear pollution. But, *mirabile dictu*, the working class has an uncanny talent for residing in polluted areas: the East End, after all, began as the location for the 'noxious trades' outside the city walls.

But to believe these inequalities are inevitable is to believe working-class children somehow need less fresh air and fewer books and smaller bedrooms. That they are in some way less human than the children born elsewhere. And to accept that, especially if you are in a position to do something about it, would require a terrible cruelty. For if we meet and touch these children, it is impossible not to feel for them. Yet their premature deaths and unnecessary (because preventable) illnesses get worse and more sharply socially divided. So our social system seems to believe that these children are somehow less human, less deserving of survival than those born to better-off parents. And that is the other side of the biblical sin of Greed, which is the sin of Pride. James Agee, writing about the Depression in the Deep South of America, called it 'a mortal sin [which] can quite as coldly and inevitably damage and wreck the human race as the most total power of "Greed" ever could' and said that 'socially, anyhow, the most dangerous form of pride is neither arrogance nor humility, but its most common denominator form, complacency'.

Still, it is necessary to go on looking after these children however much the game is rigged. And looking after children, especially little ones, is a special challenge to a doctor. A little Vietnamese mite, thin for fourteen months but with a fine high forehead, whose mother's tone of desperation on the phone makes you visit late after surgery: 'He hot. He scratch. He hot': a litany. The baby has eczema, a dry skin condition often associated with asthma. It was diagnosed, so should have been treated properly. Maybe it had been in the last bout. But now everything was wrong. Two mangy cats in the room, better than barking dogs but bad for the skin. Both parents smoking, because of the worry, a dish-sized ashtray piled high and smouldering. The child had been itching and scratching the sore parts which were lichenified and now had heavy secondary bacterial infection. The room was overheated, the blankets heavy and synthetic. Baby Nguyen was crying acutely, the sound high-pitched and inconsolable. You didn't need a thermometer, you could see his fever. The medicine box was in the kitchen, a hopeless mixture of outdated prescriptions, traditional remedies and chemist creams. The father, who delivered pizzas for a living, spoke only a little English. All the other children were awake, everybody upset by the little one's distress.

Trying to stop babies crying on night visits is ill-advised. If you fail, and you usually do, there is the ignominy of handing back a bawling baby. On the other hand, a baby in distress is a haunting, imploring, demanding sound. But as a visiting GP, you are on your own, with little back-up, equipment, or assistance, and a limited range of medicines. Try looking more carefully in the medicine carton. There is some – unused – bath emollient. 'Let's get him in a bath': it will be a chance to examine him properly and look for pustules in case it's scabies. The bath works. Somehow the tension is broken. Something is being done to the exhausted lad, even if it's only sluicing his burning thighs and face and armpits with an oily emollient. When he's settled a bit, anxious to make my exit before the next bout of crying, I give him the first sachet of an antibiotic course to eliminate the secondary infection. And a sedative suppository. They must come and see me in surgery the next day with the Chinese link worker and we'll start again.

Skin problems are demanding. Itching in young children is a singular punishment. Impossible for them to ignore. Tempting to assuage by scratching, which stimulates more histamine, which makes the itch still worse. Skin is a single continuous vital organ and its malfunctioning has immediate psychological consequences. Acne can blight adolescence; psoriasis, with its hard raised plaques and silvery exfoliation, mutilates identity. Given the vast efforts of the cosmetic industry to define beauty and sexual attraction in terms of skin care, it's not surprising that any dermatological disorders are a kind of anti-cosmetic. This applies to children, who are not yet indoctrinated, because their parents want their children to look like the perfect creatures who advertise disposable nappies. So Nguyen's mother keeps pointing at her son's face, aghast and firing away at her husband in rapid Vietnamese. Its redness and dryness, made worse by the weals of scratching, is an affront, something she has to explain away to the relatives.

So we start. The oil in the bath – yes, every bath, once a day. No bubbles or detergents. No soap any more. Soap makes the skin worse, dry and then itchy. We want to put back plenty of grease. Beth explains while I scribble diagrams of bath tubs, cross out drawings of soap bars and prescribe large pots of emollient cleansing substitutes. Now the active treatment. Steroids, once over-utilised but now often withheld mistakenly. One cream for the face, a stronger one for the body. And some medicated bandages to wrap the forearms where the infected scratching has been worse. Then we must cut back the fingernails and if necessary improvise cotton night gloves. Plan night sedation, in a dose which will need to be higher than the manufacturer's recommendation to work and will probably have the pharmacist on the phone querying it. Avoid wool and synthetics and find an Eczema Society leaflet in Vietnamese . . . some hopes. We've already been at it fifteen minutes and the mother still obviously wants something to be done *now*. A week later the infection and fever have gone but the eczema looks just as bad and the parents agitate for the hospital. Tempting. Get shot of it all to a nice paediatric skin outpatients. But not really fair: they'd probably only be back in three months' time with a scribbled bit of paper suggesting a prescription of exactly what is being used already. No translator, but the pizza man's English, under pressure, improves and we get along with a little French too. Mother still disgruntled and probably depressed. She's missed a lot of sleep; the other two girls are fed up about all the fuss the new boy is getting, and the relatives are still complaining they can't take the photos for back home. Then, a week later, the lad *is* looking better; everyone's all smiles. They thank me for being a wonderful doctor. I insist it is all their good work. Beth the

78

link worker, older and wiser than we four, smiles to be translating something positive at last. The little diagram is still there, smeared with aqueous cream and hydrocortisone.

Asthma is even more frustrating to treat. Although thought of as a disease of wheezing and shortness of breath, it is now recognised to be underdiagnosed and often presents with recurrent attacks of coughing, with three-quarters of sufferers never wheezing. It tends to get better at the age of seven, but a lot of East End children with prolonged childhood asthma go on to suffer from severe teenage bouts and adult lung disease. Even the ones that don't can lose a lot of schooltime which surprisingly quickly stunts their education; a couple of absent weeks per term can, after three years, have pulled a child down academically. And the condition is dangerous. Children can quite rapidly become distressed and start to get potentially fatal complications. And the aerosol spray treatments which are so very effective in adults can't really be used under about ten years, so inhaled powders to dilate the lungs or oral bronchodilators and anti-inflammatory drugs, which are fiddly and need careful dosing, must be used. It's a sobering test to ask patients what the medicines do, what and which is to be taken when. If they don't know, it's your fault rather than theirs. The most effective way of administering the treatment is in the form of a fine inhaled mist delivered from a nebuliser, but this is still quite an expensive piece of machinery and often goes wrong. There is the added danger that over-nebulising can mask a worsening of the asthma that really needs hospitalisation. Asthma, like its skin twin, eczema, is powerfully affected by stress and anxiety: it is often necessary to defuse emotionally a situation before treatment can begin. When housing is damp or overcrowded, when other family members are smokers, when life lacks calm and order, asthma is hard to treat effectively.

It's also a condition which it is unwise to treat by

phone advice. Parents who are familiar with the diagnosis and treatment can sometimes be overconfident and row out of their depth. On the other hand, viral upper respiratory tract infections are universal in East London all year round, spread by overcrowding, poor ventilation and repeated cross-infection, and self-limiting. But how do you know little Johnny's cough, which he's had for three weeks, isn't in fact worsening bronchospasm? Trying to assess a child's condition from a parent's tone of voice and replies over the phone is a risky business, even if a parent is known personally. One night I was quite brusque to a mother whose son had had a cough for several days but who hadn't bothered to see her own doctor within office hours. We rather grudgingly agreed she would get Calpol from the corner store and see her own GP tomorrow. And, the mandatory codicil, phone back if absolutely necessary. She did, within forty minutes while I was at another call, an old lady who had fallen and bruised but not fractured her back. It was a cold and foggy winter night and I just couldn't find the block. Thinking I remembered the way back, I parked without consulting the map, only to find, with grim fury, that it was entirely the wrong building I had skilfully approached. The right one wasn't far but required a complicated detour which left me at the wrong end of the tenement whose battered entrance lobby was graffiti-etched and sluicing with leaked water. The nebuliser slung on one shoulder, drug case in the other hand, I put down my briefcase to get the lift and remembered I had now forgotten the house number. And the lift gave no indication which floor had which numbers anyway. By the time I got to the right front door, I was in a state of suppressed fury.

But things *were* clearly going badly. The boy, about three, clad only in his vest, was panting, unable to speak because he was breathing with such desperation. His nostrils flared, torso heaved, intercostal muscles sucked in with the effort of inhalation. His head lolled and rolled backwards and forwards as his mother clutched him. All his strength was diverted to the task of breathing. The man, tall, ebony dark, was standing preoccupied and upset. His wife, young, afraid, in a summery smock dress, looked beseeching. Their respective positions, focused on the little boy, were like a nativity. But the mother had an air, too, of Porgy and Bess, something rural, something torn, something tragically out of place. The room was dark, and I dialled the hospital while examining the baby: trying to count its rapid respiratory rate whilst clinging on to the engaged signal and redialling. Why is the phone always busy when you really need them? Catfish Row; the smell of illness, their looks, my fear. Should I grab the baby and shove him in my car? Then I'm through, and a wonderful, competent medical voice is saying, 'Yes, we'll see the baby right away.' Wonderful because minutes can ebb away parked on unanswered internal hospital lines or waiting for unanswered bleeps. So competent, not because of any great experience or prowess clinically, but simply because once inside the doors of the hospital the child will be plugged into a range of resources which can intensify if its condition declines. Whereas we play a kind of clinical chess game against illness and the night.

Night-visiting children can be a terribly depressing business too. 'God bless the child,' sings Billie Holiday, 'who's got it made!' But if they haven't, even newborn babies, unblemished, open and fascinated by the world, already have their cards marked. The answering service message is cryptic: 'Callbox; baby's ill.' Of course no reply when I redial the callbox number. Who would wait at 1 a.m. at an unprotected outside phone by the Rotherhithe Tunnel? I know the buildings well, named after a pioneer socialist docker of the 1920s; they are now a squalid tenement used as short-lease temporary housing for people on the urgent homeless list. The health visitors have been fighting to open a baby clinic there but can't get a Portacabin out of the council. Most of the mothers I have met are still traumatised by their stay in the B-and-Bs. Either depressed or past caring; pissed and barely bothering to look after their un-schooled kids who at five and six years have behaviour problems galore.

The block is noisy even in the early morning. One contingent with two toddlers are leaving in a battered Cortina, and from an upstairs doorway music booms into the cold night. Phrases float into the night wrapping round the roar of the container lorries emerging from the tunnel. 'Squeeze me tight.' 'Shake your body.' 'Like wine.' Is it soca, rumba, what? There are strong smells of cooking, several cuisines, and stencilled on the lift, whose roof-fitted light is broken, is 'Nazi boss here OK'. The Cortina races off and an alsatian starts to howl. It's a zone of transition; that's what makes it so frightening, I tell myself, marching down the fifth-floor balcony. The flat is barely furnished and the baby lies on her back on the sofa crying and coughing softly. Her mother, with deep dark skin, high cheekbones, enormous, limpid eyes, is young and very beautiful even in this spartan room with its stark, ugly electric lighting. The man, older with a voice which bears the traces of education, and a shabby sports jacket, says, 'Ah, Doctor, thank you for coming.' At first it's fine: a loving trio surviving in hard times. But then I remem-ber in a blinding flash: the baby, only ten weeks old, is already on the At Risk register. Her mother, an unmar-ried Nigerian, became psychotically ill shortly after delivery and required electroconvulsive therapy. It was because the situation was so dangerous that she had been found short-term council housing. She had been simply staring at the baby for hour after hour in the hostel. But now a local alcoholic with a long criminal record, including rape, had moved in with her. Yes, there was the Tennants Extra can just nudged under the sofa. And her piercing stare wasn't lucid but incom-prehending. And his solicitude just boozy bonhomie. Or was it after all a love match which was to save and cherish that little child on the sofa? He had, after all, called a doctor. But then, was that a bruise across the face that she was trying to conceal by the odd slanting angle at which she held her head? And what, at 1 a.m., are you going to do if it is?

Thank God the baby is, despite a heavy cold, in good health. It seems a reasonable weight and (I make a foray into the kitchen) being well looked after. A coward, I start antibiotics just in case. But outside again, where there are more scurries of feet and crashing car doors, it's dizzy-making. Oddly but not impossibly, because slush money from the LDDC often coughs up incongruous grants for improvements in amenities, the central area of these godforsaken tenements is being landscaped. Two architectural students who have also ended up on the same estate told me they had had an options questionnaire. And had voted for a wooden wendy house, "Cause it will be something nice for the alkies to burn down'. Viewed from high up, the figure-of-eight patterns the yellow bulldozer has traced in the rich brown (imported) earth look like a curved ploughed field, a ludicrous rurality. Perhaps wendy houses will join sleeping policemen and 'community murals' as the stigmata of dump estates. Still, things could be worse. A young heroin and diazepam addict, whose alcoholic mother I knew, tells me the next day that she has just evicted a fellow addict on grounds of poor child care. 'She was shooting up with the baby in her arms. You don't do that, Dave.' She's reunited with her bridegroom-to-be. 'He's sticking by me now he's out. It was six days for beating me up. But I did deserve it.'

Because young children are so vulnerable, their mistreatment stirs very deep emotions. There is a long tradition in East London of local mothers resisting the interference of 'The Authorities' who descend on them from unknown worlds of competence and criticise their management of their nittie offspring. On the other hand, people have strong views about people who mistreat children: 'She's not fit to be a mother' is perhaps the strongest single East End curse, although the male equivalent is seldom heard. These mixed feelings get especially complicated in child sexual abuse. This is higher than average in Tower Hamlets, although it is not evenly spread and tends to occur more in the lumpen white areas than the more mixed and cosmopolitan zones. Although not much recorded by doctors in the older days, it probably existed more as attempts at incestuous slap and tickle after a heavy night in the pub than interference with younger children, since working men then took very little part in child care. But the high level of male unemployment and the consequent softening of strict sexual divisions of labour mean men are more often with pre-pubertal girls.

Seeing one's first sexually damaged child's vagina or sodomised anus is as much a milestone in a doctor's career as passing Finals, and is far more upsetting than even the ghoulish rites of post-mortem with the bloody circular saw and splintered sternums. Medical students are hardened, supposedly, with demonstrations of X-rays of people who fed wires attached to car batteries into their bladder for fun, or who stuff jars of cold cream up their anus on Fridays. But self-inflicted injuries, however bizarre, and accidents, however terrifying, even rape, somehow don't upset so much as the physical abuse of the very young. For what is so disorientating is that the victim is *so* trapped, not just physically in the home but emotionally too (it is her father or his stepfather) and so, denying, often presents sideways with withdrawal and depressive signs or sometimes sexual precocity. Given that diagnosis is tenuous (small children don't usually lie about sexual encounters, but finding a way for them to be able to talk freely and reliably is difficult), the clinical assessment of CSA is difficult. The physical signs are not clear-cut or agreed. And apparent from intra-departmental rivalries, the potential for problems is worsened by the fact that the allegation, it has been swiftly discovered, can be an effective weapon in a custody dispute. My experience, which is thankfully small, would suggest that, apart from the truly psychopathic male, the majority are step-father-daughter cases in homes already in a state of social disorganisation and sexual breakdown, a sort of rape-in-the-family. But what is more disturbing is the extent of the emotional consequences. Because of the bravery of the doctors who first reported to a disbelieving public the scale of this problem, it is now possible for more and more grown-up women to come to terms with their own abuse. It has turned out to be a powerful element in so many cases of adult depression, attempted suicide and sexual malfunction, that the self-hatred and despair engendered by it deserve to be taken with extreme seriousness, even if the allegation is ambiguous.

So often it comes back to alertness when performing the routine development checks. The syndromes which need to be identified as early as possible, either to remedy them or to allow the parents to plan for them. The sickly baby who is persistently below expected weights, perhaps because of undiagnosed asthma or renal problems, perhaps because of either deliberate or accidental mismanagement. The mother or father who is finding the going hard, or is isolated or sinking under the continuing demands of child care, running a home and paying the bills. And, perhaps, the kiddy who is being abused by beloved dad.

In all these fields there is not the slightest doubt that single mothers have a harder time. The idea that living on child benefit and Social Security with an unnamed father would prove a route of female emancipation was far-fetched in the early 1970s when the real value of welfare was far higher. The single mother in the East End nowadays is more likely to have got pregnant young by accident and have a boyfriend who, if still around, is happy to take credit for and play with the child from time to time, but who also has other girl-friends and perhaps other children. Or an older woman may well have chosen to leave an unhappy or violent relationship, often after a period in a Women's Aid centre, and does not want the father to have access. Others might have a husband or boyfriend who is 'away': enjoying the hospitality of Her Majesty. Certainly there is sometimes strong solidarity between single mothers both sharing and standing together. And this echoes the traditional East End 'matrilocal' communities where women would publicly gang up not only against the landlord and the bailiff but against errant husbands and boyfriends. And it marks modern East End women's desire for sexual relationships with emotional intimacy and sexual choice rather than the utilitarian and unromantic deal so often parodied in the music-hall songs, whereby 'He' brings home the wages (minus drink money) and she, in turn, makes house and puts up with intercourse.

In the old East End, sexual antagonism was acknowledged. The women were tough and entitled to violence if the man didn't deliver his wages. Men would expect the women to be entirely responsible for household sustenance and care and clothing of the children, and woe betide her if dinner wasn't on the table. Both enjoyed rowdy weekend drinking. And elements of these patterns persisted through the postwar prosperity when sociologists argued that the traditional working-class extended family had been largely replaced by a middle-class 'nuclear' structure. But perhaps the 'single mother' with sole responsibility for looking after the house and bringing up the children is really a traditional East End figure. Only now she depends on the state rather than a husband for regular income and can choose which men she admits to her life and when. But the price of such independence is often impoverishment and exhaustion.

Married or single, black or white, the real needs of East End parents and children are strikingly consistent. And uncannily echo the demands of the 1920s when Poplar, London's first Labour borough with a strong contingent of women councillors, began the construction of the modern welfare state. They are therefore hardly unreasonable in the late twentieth century. Better maternity services with more convenience and personal choice and the end of the hospital antenatal cattle market which means an afternoon's waiting for an examination which takes five minutes. Accessible baby clinics with cheap good-quality baby food. Good-quality, reliable, collective under-five care and well-equipped, well-staffed nursery schools. Adequate financial support for full-time mothers of young children. Better housing with children's needs taken into consideration and the right of a council place for all young families. An environment which is friendly to young children: clean, safe and cheerful. Proper local facilities for recreation and relaxation. And employers who cater for childbirth by allowing adequate maternity arrangements, flexible working hours and crèche facilities.

What modern East End mothers get is another matter. The combination of cuts in the hospital services and sheer weight of numbers clogs up the maternity clinics which suffer from high staff turnover and consequent low morale. The sole female consultant pushing community antenatal care was suspended for eighteen months on what proved to be trumped-up charges by her male colleagues. As the Royal College of Midwives reported in February 1990, mortality rates among the newborn are beginning to increase again in Tower Hamlets and other inner city areas and the mortality rates overall compare unfavourably with many European countries. Under-five facilities are exceptionally poor even by the low British standards: there are some self-organised or church-run One O'Clock clubs, but pre-school education, vital for children and parents, where it exists is private, starting price £90 a week, and facilities poor. The local authority services are overrun: Poplar Play Centre, for example, opened in 1986, has a waiting list of 180, and the small number of social service nursery places have to be reserved for children 'at risk' or in very special need, essentially supervision units rather than nurseries. At school age, 600 Tower Hamlets over-five-year-old children are awaiting admission to school, their constitutional right. Once there, reception classes often contain thirty or more children. To hear each child read individually once would take two and a half hours minimum out of an effective teaching day of four hours. How much time does that leave for the ten subjects of the national curriculum, or for the kids with language, physical, mental, or behavioural needs, or for the teacher to update the 300 written progress records? And how on earth will Tower Hamlets, which has relied on heavy subsidy from the old ILEA, finance an adequate local education service on a son-of-poll tax which a large number of residents can't or won't pay? This when the 1990 annual report by Her Majesty's Inspectors already concludes that 'there are serious problems of low and under-achievement, of poor teaching and inadequate provision'. The Tower Hamlets social services are now under formal investigation for inadequacies in their children's homes and children's services and the local schools are increasingly staffed by teachers from Holland and New Zealand.

As for a guaranteed maternal income, the real value of Child Benefit, the one payment which goes straight to the mother, is reduced every year by the Party of the Family, and the allowances like Family Credit and Income Support are means-tested. Female unemployment in Tower Hamlets is one of the highest in London and in such circumstances even large-scale employers, like the NHS, need make no effort about workplace crèches. Pregnancy is still effectively grounds for dismissal in many small firms or for part-time workers. Since the abolition of the GLC many voluntary ethnic and specialist groups providing help for children have had to close and some of the fine play facilities, for example, in the centre of Victoria Park, opened under their auspices, are deteriorating. Against the grim backdrop of urban decline, housing crisis and economic recession, the efforts of doctors or health visitors can make only very limited improvements. What is remarkable is how well East End mothers do themselves in conditions which would tax better-off and better educated mothers. But how much better things would be if they and their children were allowed to flourish without the incessant erosion of economic and social deprivation. We have progressed in absolute terms but those advances have not been made available equitably across the board. 'When one knows of the conditions of life,' wrote John Scurr in 1924, 'one stands in admiration of the struggle which is put up against their environment by thousands of men and women. . . . What chance have they or their children. . . . Our society passes them by and abuses them for [what] our social system has thrust upon them.'

CHAPTER 6

---◦◦◉◦◦---

VISITATIONS

Called out to a horribly grinning child who was said to be ill. The disgruntled mother shouts, 'You call me a liar' at it. Who's the problem?

Meeting with community psychiatric nurses. We deal in quick succession with eleven-year-old glue-sniffers, multiple incest, persistently violent father, epileptic mother refugee from battered wives' home, high anxiety mothers, absent fathers, unhappy marriages, disturbed children. A doctor nodded off on his examination couch; is it tiredness or inviolability? In three years I am at his funeral.

Called to a twenty-year-old by her mother who complains about delay. 'She could have died while I'm on the phone.' Not a good start. On arrival, mother radiates insecurity and rage in equal quantities, smoking so hard she can hardly talk. The sister perches herself coquettishly on the sink rim. The patient, heavily made up, is fully dressed under the covers. Complaining of a 'lump that had gone down inside'. Examination difficult as she only reluctantly removes her underwear and then only outer layers. She's twenty weeks pregnant. She grins triumphantly, inanely. NF stickers promising 'a black future' on top of the stairs.

Antenatal clinic in Hackney; only 'white' mother of the afternoon a nineteen-year-old Irish lass who is thin as a rake, marigold-haired and has a face like a crucifix. The others are a cheerfully polyglot mixture of Jamaican, Egyptian, Turkish, Sikh. Anarchist punk comes late dressed like a disintegrating tea cosy. Doesn't want to be examined. The woman consultant, strict and kindly, is distressed by the fact that so few of her patients are either married or Christian. The Turkish lady is lost in fear, pain and apprehension; her more experienced friend announces to me knowingly, 'She don't know what's coming.' The punk is enormously constipated. Boots holed and voluminous clothes smell of corporate squatting. Clinic walls have pictures of vegetables and eggs, useful ingredients of diet. 'Are you on a good diet?' the consultant asks. 'No, I don't want to lose weight.'

'I live in a block with fifty houses. There's only three men who don't wear a turban. Myself and an Irishman and an Egyptian,' says Edward Farthing. This is not true. But he has said it many times.

Out-of-date tattoos and cracked knuckles. Heroin . . . which means lost fathers, painful migrations, blocked veins and a succession of changes of address. Wants a letter for the court. Again.

In the top of a tower block a Rembrandt lady, diabetic, sits with her daughters staring down at the muddy Thames but not seeing it. Her face in the long afternoon light is clear, high-boned, parchment-coloured. Her urine eeks down a translucent tube which coils to a flat bag on the floor. A spiral of urine is slowly corrugating inside the bag. The family watch her silently. A portrait of static depression. Lift says 'Lansbury rules'. Not George any more. An end of something that's about to go but never does. Against the mud, the LDDC skyscrapers glint. In 1990 this block, Risby House, was demolished for the Docklands motorway.

Christmas home visits. Alka Seltzer and warm loathing. Pass print union picket line at Wapping; the union full-timers are putting out the fires (literally). Baby cheered up by new arrival, bored by his circumstances. Exit strewn with litter and four or five supermarket trolleys buggering each other. Lift's surfaces tattoed with mis-spelt swearwords. Christmas wrapping and food packs blow up and down the corridors of concrete gloom. One flat made derelict full of broken machinery and rubble. In the corner broken mirrors and smashed reproduction portraits of big-eyed children that East Enders like. On way out, a cheerful pair stagger in: their fumes ignitable. A mess with people left to fight and love and laugh it out.

A boy with stomach pain at 1 in the morning. Eventually decide he had eaten too much and proved right by prodigious vomiting over my trousers. Enter Teviot, ghoulish, low-rise corridors, past a smashed mountain bike, newish, as if masticated by giant jaws. Big graffiti: 'Beware. You Are Entering The Teviot Estate' which no-one has bothered to paint out. This one's probably only gastric flu but in view of the empty one-litre vodka bottle in the inbuilt bar may be dehydrated for other reasons. Then called about a baby which had been crying for four hours. It has 'just settled' by the time I arrived.

Flu epidemic: headaches, fever, sweats, but people are rather disappointed if you tell them that's all they've got. Would they prefer malaria? Two burst eardrums, both thin emaciated women, straggly hair, blood at external meatus, who have endured a lot of beating before this latest blow. Scabies and lice commonplace even in the clean and neat. Worms too. Child consti-pated for four days; on rectal exam extract a crab-apple-sized faecal mass. He stops crying, family wondrous. A small miracle performed.

In the last week I have seen four male alcoholics under twenty-five. Manual workers delivered by the sack, the dole, or family crisis, to the drink. One says it's the pain of an NHS-postponed hernia which led him to guzzle Bacardi. Others talk grudgingly about marriages gone, jobs lost, temporary housing, children who don't care.

'The Nose' is different: twenty-one and quite happy with a dose of gonorrhoea from a prostitute. Gravitated to Limehouse: lives alone in rudimentary bed-sit. Transfers price tags from beer cans to wine in Asda and gets them quarter price. Convinced his nose was the world's mockery so driven himself into isolation; quite a high risk of suicide.

The next a barman who eventually concedes his stomach pains and weight loss might be to do with drinking one and a half bottles of whisky a day.

Then a 'record producer' who said he needed sleepers because he'd been attacked by black men in a white Mercedes, and that his wife had gone with his best friend. Would send our staff a selection of free records for being so kind. But didn't live at the given temporary address, not known at work. No free records ever came. Fugue, fraud, or alcohol.

Mr Ryan had been drinking whisky and beer in bouts since sixteen: angel cheeks, fresh face, blue eyes, carrot hair, a Tralee colour scheme. Three days later in the medical ward withdrawing, he has tremors and hallucinates toads grazing on his torso.

Alcohol is cheap, alcoholism a liquid correlative of recession and unemployment, the old London drunkenness, a numbing you can now purchase at the supermarket. All four were joyless. At least the pub drunkards possessed a kind of delight.

Bradford Asian couple in their teens: he Hendrix-

headed, she almond-faced, have run away. Had a fight
with parents who found out she had had an abortion.
He then overdosed (quite seriously). She slashed her
wrists (less seriously) by his hospital bed. Now OK.
'Happy?' he says in thick Brum. 'I'm so 'appy I've
brought her some flowers.' They are gentle to each
other: idyllic now such sudden beauty.

Mr Waller, ex-docker. 'Downloader', went into hold
with hook and ropes. Fruit, refrigerated meat, veg.,
nuts from Beirut, Damascus and Limassol. Via barge
or bogies into the sheds and bays until the Covent
Garden lorries picked them up. In turn reloaded boats
with old axles, scrap metal, machinery. Registered here
since 1916, born in the surgery road. Moved to Stepney, then Bow, then back to Rhodeswell Road according to ascent up housing ladder. Now has pernicious
anaemia, skin with a citrus gleam.
    Also woman obsessed by her desire for sexual events:
a female Casanova. Another woman, acute anxiety,
mothering son and husband. Then cross they can't
stand up for themselves. Thin girl who turns out to
have been a prostitute in Rugby of all places. 'Open the
door less,' I say. 'Try shielding yourself from men.'
Flotsam and jetsam: the female foot-soldiers of mental
illness. Nothing grand, just everyday sadness.

Childbirth a combination of endless waiting and then
near panic. Exhorting straining pudendas to unleash
their offspring. Slow torment of dilation then released
into pushing. Head see-saws round the birth canal,
stretching the perineum like a round-roofed circus tent.
The baby is pink as an inner tube and slippery-slimy.
Mother's disbelief, just before delivery close to some
sort of death, then exhilaration, the head soars free and
then twists and the rest, shoulders and body, is easy.
Earlier, as baby's skull descended past the rectum, a
tiny squiggle of faeces anointed the spot where the baby
is to land. The baby sometimes stains the liquor with

its own faeces, called meconium. So one enters this world clad in shared shit and blood, screaming and crying at the same time.

Warm, cosy, chaotic winter. A hospital porter comes in with a pulled back: he's been lifting so many corpses, the cost of a spell of cold weather. 'The fridges were full. Twenty or more. Some so bent up they wouldn't fit the trays. Tried to flatten one old girl out and did my back.'

Visit surgical ward in hospital to see a patient. Didn't recognise him. Lost stones. Eyes gleaming out of a threadbare face. Normally a quiet man. Now angry: about the conditions of the wards, the workload of the nurses. 'Wards *are* dirty. They should have diagnosed me earlier. The bastards. The government. I wish they could have something really nasty happen to them and spend three weeks in here. They wouldn't talk all that crap about the NHS being OK.' Wants to retire to his sister's. But there are no jobs out there; she has little money. He has no savings. 'I'm nothing, am I? Only a caretaker.' A very bitter death.

At 2.30 a.m. tossing and turning. Phone goes. 'She's in pain and I can vouch for that.' An apparently stoic husband about his spouse's agonising back pain. Down the motorway, up the flats' steps. Rubbish-strewn, washing line, broken Campari bottles. Woman is fifty, looks seventy, falling over pissed. Chest sounds like bubbles blown through soup. Pleuritic rub harsh as emery paper. Diamorphine stat. Room cross between a caravan and cave: dank and dirty and rich in old smells.

Weekend on call. Baby girl with sudden swelling, knees drawn up, crying, and impossible to examine. Father doesn't acknowledge me, staring fixedly at the TV snooker. As if he's nothing to do with it. Then on and on: kids with stomach pain, babies vomiting, Vietnamese family huddled in an old docker's flat, two families sharing food, sixteen altogether. Rice served from two-foot-high plastic tubs. The men watching Canadian ice hockey, commentary in French. Sick baby three years old, neurologically retarded from birth. Beautiful slack baby bounced mechanically on the knee of his smartly dressed mother to show me she cared. Like a doll. Then directed upstairs to the Buis' flat, full of electronic items, and another chest infection. Much multiple translation, my French to their Cantonese. Try to explain that my stethoscope can't stop the coughing.

Then to lady of ninety-six who has just died. Already stiffening as family slowly assemble round the bed, formally like a wedding photo in a developing tank. Devout: the incense, nicotine. The older sister devastated; her mortality ablaze. Considerate district nurse, her blue uniform makes formal the loss. Me respectful of a body I never knew but will see again in a galvanised box in the undertaker's. After I sign the cremation form, a shifty man gives me £18 cash in a dirty brown envelope. I see him later chainsmoking in the cafe and obsessionally playing the fruit machine. Save us from dodgy undertakers.

Long walk, past blocked-off roads. Glad it's daylight. Passing into an infinity of coughing children. Husband cuts off. Says nothing except 'Goodbye, mate' as I leave. Cystitis: acute. Infected eczema; 'Is it catching?'
    Fifteen visits, two admissions later, at 2 a.m. go to see sixteen-year-old Nigerian boy with the looks of a male model and stomach pain. Fuss plus plus, unimpressive. Get called back two hours later. Admit. It settles immediately. Who knows?

In Peking restaurant LDDC executives are parcelling up the docklands' visual vistas for advertising clients. Arguing about percentages. 'We'll supply everything:

film, catering, birds.' Getting drunker and noisier. 'Let's get bottom line on this. If you were me, what would you be thinking?' 'The world's your oyster here in Docklands. We run things. When we got your letter, our first reaction was, send in the heavy mob. Kick 'em. Then the more liberal among us said, let's talk to them, we can screw 'em afterwards.' Gangsters in pinstripes.

Ex-docker is a depressive, addicted to tranquillisers. Devoured by his own hopelessness which dates from the death of his only daughter in car accident. A year earlier she had been left by her husband with four children, who subsequently went into care, place unknown. Simultaneous death of his own mother from a painful spleen cancer which required interminable blood transfusions. He has a diarrhoea which no one can explain except as a result of his neurosis.

Next a boozer with 'Love' and 'Hate' tattooed on knuckles, stigmata of the Belfast-Glasgow-Teesside lumpen of the industrial crucifixion. Lugged in by goal-post of a Salvationist. Uncontrolled for nearly twelve years: wine, sherry, Special Brew. 'Anything I can lay my hands on, as early in the day as I can, pissed for breakfast.'

The next a portly Cockney. Lots of chat, could be minicab controller or barrow boy but 'wants help' with heroin; forearms tracked as if sewing machines have been up and down them. He uses his groin and ankle veins too. Also speed and booze. Eleven convictions and coming up for his twelfth: the only reason he's here.

Then baby gastroenteritis or rather parental anxiety. Hard-to-control blood pressure, a West Indian nurse. Hop-picking Cockney with bladder cancer. Hospital cleaner now contracting for her own job, at reduced wages, 'cracking up', unable to work at the speed she was now supposed to and do the job properly. Doing the job properly matters to her. Reported to the supervisor for 'chatting to the patients'! A quartet of tiny Glaswegian kids, all way below the weight charts, all on the At Risk register. But the case conference is cancelled due to staff shortages. Allowed no toys. 'They'd only break them.' Parents cheerfully incompetent rather than vicious, except when drunk. Then security dog-handler who works twenty-hour shifts guarding LDDC. Got thrown out of home with a court order to stay away from his kids. Takes a Valium before he goes into action with his dog who is the calmer of the two. Police station cleaning lady moans about the endless police parties. 'No wonder they can't arrest anyone, they're too pissed.'

Ex-docker, austere man, well regarded, with a lump that at first could have been a hernia; turned out to be inoperable Ca. His wife comes separately to cry, careful to avoid him. 'Tell him it's all right': a kind lie which gets harder. 'I didn't realise what people go through. And how you people do your job. And that good things can come out of bad.'

Another man dying was a captain, eyes slightly mid-distance as if still alert to maritime danger. He sits in a darkened room protected from the pain by morphine, nodding off, alert only with effort. Wears neat short-sleeved shirts with shipshape buttoned pockets. His many children, busy, jovial, despairing, are in the kitchen corridor. 'How long's he got, Doc?' His daughter hopes he will 'talk', that is, break down, share, face it together. 'But he's not that sort of man. None of them were. He couldn't tell me because he's closest to me. He'll tell one of the boys.' He doesn't. He goes off to the hospice eventually. His daughter and I help him step up to the ambulance but he goes on his own with a piercing farewell glance. They arrange to get the local church opened up for the funeral. A telephone rings, unanswered, throughout the eulogy. He had been christened and married here. Fullbodied singing of

VISITATIONS

'There is a green hill far away'. The churchyard is double-parked with black BMWs and Sierras.

Old depressed lady, disinhibited, spends all day masturbating herself and cursing at passers-by. Admit another lady dying and regret it, the awful last ambulance ride. But her daughter had been sleeping in the same room for months: things were too intense by the end.

Summer in East London, people near-naked and caked in sweat, dust, sun lotion and diesel fumes. The more outdoor the more generous, the more open and less ill. Balmy at night, erotic, full of chance.

Old man in dirty clothes neglecting himself. Braces and TV. Three strokes and awaiting his fourth. Toothless wife. Then high-rise flat awash with babies and mothers and cigarette smoke, overheated, cheerful pandemonium. No one concentrating, children either ignored or shouted at. Therefore always demanding and unruly.

Back pain at midnight. Single seventeen-year-old in squat. Beside bed a signed photo. Not her boyfriend, a male stripper she had met the previous night. Virtually no possessions but emerged each morning in immaculate eye make-up and leather miniskirt. She'd fallen over in her mayonnaise factory. Says she works in puddles of pickle juice and oil. Later her child goes into care because of heroin. Looked after a woman dealer's dogs and got paid in heroin. 'But I shopped her, the cow.' She comes back occasionally, after dihydrocodeine.

Patients with high anxiety, low expectations. Exhibitionists: wrist-slashers, plate-throwers, overdose artists. Manic depressive with his bits of paper. Grandiose. High pressure of language: rictus smiles. Odd, unmatching clothes (sign of Sally Army). Rants off slamming the door. Demented old lady with flat but

99

no carpets, cupboards but no food and a fire that was singeing her stockings, aroma of corned beef, piss and scorched nylon. Full of fury: at the relatives who had 'deserted' her, the social worker and me. Could hide in the psychiatric highways and byways of the old NHS. Now slung back to 'the community', the sociological equivalent of Siberia. URTI, ulcerative colitis, booze, pregnancy, TB, stroke, depressed, diabetic, ear, sick boy, 'pains all over'. And housing: 'Can't stand it no longer, what you going to do, Doc?' If the road to heaven is paved with housing letters, sainthood is guaranteed.

Not dirt or 'squalor' but low horizons, cut-off options, numbing of possibility. Clamber round lifts and get lost in hardboard annexes: sectors of walled sub-city. But the quirkiness or warmth or humanity or stupidity or sheer fecklessness of people still raise the heart. Two huge Fellini ladies in nighties pirouette in to assist my examination of knee of a man in oil-streaked boiler suit: a strange ballet. Despite their weight they move gracefully, as if sub-aqua.

The nights can be comic too. When a dog nips you as you examine a sleeping child supposed to be inconsolable. Or you drop the lubricated sterile catheter on the filthy floor and the cat nabs it. Or lady after massive stroke, approaching death like a train into a tunnel, and they say, 'What are you going to do about it, Doctor?' And bellow: 'Pull yourself together, Mum' at the corpse-to-be.

When it's bright at night, you can imagine Limehouse between the wars: bright lights, sailors and foreign cargo. The majesty of briny wind across the Blue Bridge to the choppy flatness of dockwater.

New patients with impossible demands, old faces with familiar problems. Batty girl: 'The paper in my head tells me to love you.' Entering odd, gloomily lit areas of social disorganisation, homes where logic seems to have gone missing. Bare room: bar fire, meter, TV; many high-heeled shoes, about forty pairs! 'Keeping the vodka to one bottle a day, Doc,' she says and falls over. Her handbag clanks. Next call, meet a man on the stairs. He says, 'Are you the doctor?' I say, 'Are you the patient?' He's been dragged out of the pub to meet me.

Possible miscarriage in thigh-length Afghan coat. Not sure if she's pregnant; always manages to miss the Pill the night of a reconciliation with old flame. Is it an ectopic? Thrashing epileptic with children cowering in the mess of vomit and broken sofa. He's drunk too. Neighbours won't open their door to let me use the phone. Beneath him is a piece of crumpled paper on which is scrawled 'One beef curry and rice. One prawn balls. Two crackers. One mixed vegetables. Six lagers. One bottle of sweet wine. With all my love Darling XXX. Then you might be pregnant after that.' A lumpen proletarian love poem. Then a shingles lady who shows me round her bottled analgesics like a curator of antiquities. Her room is hung with old furnishings, lacks ventilation, a lingering presence of gas, staleness and scouring powder.

Cheerful anarcho-feminist squatter running health food shop who wants a home delivery because she 'hates hospitals'. But thinks bailiffs are coming. Ethiopian seaman joined by pregnant wife twenty years younger. Their baby has six fingers on the left hand which he wants to keep: 'Allah's good luck sign.'

Someone proudly throws across the table the Valium he's managed to stop taking. They land on a piece of paper where I have just drawn a diagram of a prostate gland.

101

Mad actors. Pregnant painters. Drunken sailors. A stonemason with a 'Tear here' tattoo at the throat. A widow talks about the death. He'd gone off for radiotherapy. Come home. Felt ill. She'd put him into bed. He'd coughed blood, gasped and then was dead. She recalled the moment of death with a certain luminosity: as people do. Then the daughter who had lost a baby but been able to hold it cries too.

Of fifteen patients, three have waiting list problems, which they complain about with various degrees of anger and insight. Vietnamese man possibly a bit psychotic living with his elderly father in a barrack room. From Hue. Fisherman, florist, tailor, thief. East London occupations for 500 years. Visit a vast Nigerian glowing with procreation. While her men play cards and boil rice in the front room, she undresses and oils a gleaming baby.

It's election day and the Labour candidate sits lunching with agent, eating Chinese sweets, not very urgent. 'Been addicted to ginger since I was a girl,' says the candidate. 'In the old days the Labour Party could run an election in their sleep; they don't understand a good canvass nowadays.' A man from the LDDC bursts in with bottles of champagne he wants to put in the fridge for his son's evening birthday meal.

Back at the old people's home I certify the death of a nice old gentleman whose mother had been a flower-seller in Piccadilly and died of gin. Always wore a trilby. Psychiatric crises. Manic depressive: manic as fireworks after only two weeks, an epileptic ex-BM candidate with a leucotomy who's either overdone her medication or just passed out with the effort of it all. Lots of Vietnamese today: Dungs, Buis, Ngs and Tuongs. Of the 16,000 refugees accepted by Britain in 1981, only 3,600 were settled in London but many more gravitated back to the capital. The British Refugee

Council's early efforts faltered: learning English is the key but a difficult one to turn. There was no indigenous London Vietnamese community (as there would have been in France) and established Chinese community was initially resentful. See them shopping in supermarkets (because you don't have to ask) and looking at a lot of TV, not understanding very well. Another case conference where child conceived, concealed, delivered, rejected (because the wrong colour) by mother, father told it was dead anyway (by social worker), adopted, retrieved (by penitent parent), lost (in pub during celebratory spree), readopted. Not much of a start in life.

Hackney is skips, Indian takeaways and estate agents. Tower Hamlets is video shops, alsatians and traffic jams. Punks trying to prise off the front of soon-to-be yuppified apartments. There is a fight at the checkout. Mother breaks down: exhausted by child care. Demoralised by marriage. Imprisoned by home. Salesman elongating sickness for financial reasons. Ears to be syringed. Temp patient who has delusions and recently attempted suicide. Severely subnormal couple who should be in care but run away . . . need wardship order. Taking a smear when patient says, 'Could you arrange detox for my boyfriend: he wants to come off.' Girlfriend is ex-heroin, now sedative-dependent. Bears scars and bruises of beatings–up.

Tired: because up at 6.30 a.m. trying to comfort the bereaved and at 6.30 at night still visiting a Calor-gas-heated Bangladeshi squat. Last weekend a Hackney tower block demolished: a great public celebration. Little plumes from the window, then the entire structure gives a great cough and drops downwards and inwards amid rumble and cheers. Nothing whatsoever wrong with tower blocks themselves: what's wrong is jerry-built, cheapskate, maintenance-less, amenity-desolate tower blocks. The popular triumph at their

demise a Hackney equivalent to demolishing Stalin stat-
ues in Eastern Europe.

This week's 'Temporary Patients':

I.v. heroin 4 years £30 per day wants night sedation. Doesn't listen. Just wants scrip.

Genital herpes.

Lump builder with pulled shoulder.

Gay man with puritus ani.

Bereaved can't sleep.

'Drying out' died later.

Epileptic with angina.

Letter about psoriasis for linen grant. 'No longer
available.'

Chinese man dying of cancer. All his family seem to
loathe him. Candid at least. Daughter has acute shellfish
allergy. He's under a blanket being shouted at by his
wife. Desolate travellers' site: smashed TVs and burnt
sofas. Cooking smells and kids' clothes on the line.
Wooden fence used as toilet: faeces and urine. Hospital
porter can't sleep because he's got industrial sewing
machines pounding away next door. 'My block's
becoming a sweatshop.' The men who collect the
women's clothes drive new BMWs. Ends up by buying
into a posh apartment and splits up with girlfriend
about the rent. So it's a good thing he didn't tell the
council he was moving out. People let out anger on
you. A weight off their mind is now on yours.

Five visits after midnight after a day of consultations,
inquiries, recriminations and visits. Next day the lefties
are going under. Aspirant rock-star from St Albans
who's slumming it and cracks up. Messenger who is
kipping on friends' floor and trying to organise a bikers'

union. Feminist health food communes which break down in debt.

When resolve to nurse at home collapses there are recriminations. 'Dad, do you want to go into hospital?' and when the old boy took a breath, 'See, I told you, Doc,' says upset daughter in tight jeans and fag. The other daughter with suit sits fuming, handbag on lap. She's the Billericay one.

Baby-faced heroin addict from Bootle. Scally clothing, arm full of tracks. Been in prison several times. 'I keep moving.' Drunken prostitute mother whose son is going into care, abused by one of her alcoholic boy-friends. Foster-home staff profess to be concerned in case they catch Aids from him. The managers send memo on the political economy of paper clips.

Tall sad Somalian. 'Husband in bush.' Alone in estate named after left-wing docker. Her son tries to explain euphemistically: 'Can't have no more.' She needs ter-mination, raped it seems by compatriot. She already has acid reflux. 'No more fried food,' I end. 'Fried food, fried food, fried food,' she says, laughing and holding her belly.

Cough and cold phones at 2 a.m. 'for reassurance'. Remains of dinner on the floor being eaten by dogs when I visit. Half-dressed dirty children. Mother young but lines of pain and age already round her eyes. Hus-band has flamboyant drinking bouts during which he injures himself and others. Tries and tries again for mechanical jobs. She is scared to run away, scared to stay. Can't tell anyone in case he found out. Flat not in her name. Child bemused while mother cries and sobs.

Talk to an ex-docker, trade unionist, now a little deaf. 'I'd like the TV to show what LDDC have done to this area where there has been so much money made and

105

so much money spent to so little benefit.' Let us all sing together the Hymn to Human Greed. We are governed by grasping philistines, that's understandable. I just wish they didn't pretend to be moral as well.

Pulls out list of the noises the noisy kids have made. Wants stronger sleeping pills. Robbed, no insurance. Also smashed car; adds, 'I was quite pissed at the time.'

'Blacks Superior' crossed out: 'Go home'.

Menopausal depression, sweats. 'Usually tired. Always got a cough. Well, I smoke, don't I. Feel like I'm fading away.'

The reality of sudden death: husband with tummy pain. Felt better. Went out to the kitchen. Dropped dead.

'I'm going mad,' 'I'm going mad,' a litany.

Noise: in the streets, the sirens, car noise.

Middle-aged lady with nerves. Husband's confused, embarrassed. Stocky, robust. Stands as if he has been in the army.

Mr Abrahams the presser has a cough. 'I get plenty of steam at work.'

Old addicts, subservient, looking like bank clerks used to. Tough constitution; survived septicaemias, pneumonias, even tubercle.

Old Irish builder's labourer, well held, open face. A Catholic trade unionist, he's from an age when young women were called Vera and said 'Lord Luv A Duck' and Irishmen were wild and handsome. He courted Becky Silverman, the Jewish communist. But he's 'not political'. Comes in to tell you the boxing results. 'Call me a bastard.' Just hates the bosses. Becky's always cheerful. 'Twenty-five years before I got married and then I chose a wrong 'un,' she jokes. Always steadfast smile. Just like Mrs Levy, who married a Chinese chef from Brick Lane and whose sons are Telecom engineers. 'Money? All the money gets spent after you've done the rent.'

Alf Logan, a skilled fitter, sacked. 'Best thing I've done

in the last six months is make a doll's house for my granddaughter. Now I'm fixing the neighbour's invalid chair with fibre glass.' He's from Bow, a bit posh; Bethnal Green is somewhat shady; Poplar tough men and fierce wives.

In Bethnal Green, they say, 'Repulsive what them doctors do. Gave me stuff that smelt of cat's piss.' There was a doctor in Bow used to say, 'I'm a married man, you're a married woman. We both know you don't go to bed to play dominoes.' His second wife gave him some dominoes on his wedding night.

CHAPTER 7

LESS ELIGIBLE

After forty years of trying, rather slowly, to build a welfare state, and ten years of rather more rapid attempts to replace it with a social market, poverty is widespread and growing in Britain. Our welfare standards now fall below those set in other European nations to which we regard ourselves as economically superior.

Poverty, of course, is a very relative thing. Today's poor certainly have more purchasing power than those in the Great Depression of the 1930s. The modern UB40 can afford to keep a pet, watch a video, even order a takeaway. But they still lack what the employed worker takes for granted: a regular holiday, domestic privacy, variety in diet and the ability and the means to go out in the evenings and weekends. Malnutrition is not nowadays a matter of starvation but more often poor-quality, over-sweet, filling food which is liable to cause obesity. Poor housing means chronic overcrowding and loss of privacy, a compulsory communalism which manufactures neurosis rather than roofs falling in. For, far from being a decade of genuine prosperity, the 1980s consumer boom has had a very limited effect on the real quality of life in East London and unemployment and thus poverty become the fate not just of the single, the ill and the socially isolated, but of fit and previously well-employed working-class families. Improved living standards for the better-off have not 'trickled down' to working-class families. Instead, families on supplementary benefit are now worse off compared with the rest of the population. The number of children living in poverty, below or around the supplementary benefit level, has doubled, thousands more are homeless and inequalities in health and education have widened.

This was the inevitable result of social policies which deliberately reversed the trend, lethargic but long-term, towards a more equal distribution of wealth and which have sought to run down and privatise the provisions of the welfare state. The philosophy of economic liberalism rested on the idea that if humans and businesses really compete against each other with as little intervention, regulation, or welfare as possible, a new efficient world will reconstitute itself, phoenix-like, out of the ashes of those who don't make it. Thus, out of the dismay and debris of East London's traditional manual trades and social services will come, hey presto, the renaissance at Canary Wharf. The reality was somewhat different, as the history of the late nineteenth century in East London would have predicted. Without safety regulation, labour protection and trade unionism, manual workers are at the mercy of employers who do as they will and have a pool of casual replacements to which to turn. Without a clear social policy on land tenure and public housing, the urban poor will either be exploited by landlordism or have great difficulty finding anywhere of their own to live as they grow up and want to leave their family home. And the lives of the old, the sick, the single parent will disintegrate without a reasonable level of support whose buying power is consistent with the wages of the employed. Without these provisions on which the postwar welfare consensus depended, the other vices of cities – crime, homelessness, penury, beggary and physical decay – supervene.

Of course, a great deal more is necessary to make modern city life enjoyable: good public transport, egalitarian, progressive education services, the space and the physical facilities to enjoy good health, the means to experience culture. But in the East End such refinements do not begin to exist: there is no cinema or theatre now open in the entire borough of Tower Hamlets; 600 schoolchildren are barred from schools through lack of teachers; over a thousand families are registered as homeless; and the cultural amenities are the pub or the video. Indeed, the provision of a place to live and a job to do, something that Elizabethan East London could probably muster, are today, at the end of a prolonged boom which rebuilt the commercial city, under question. The 'classless' society' where the social good is pursued rationally is, in reality, an incoherent edifice without logic or equity, a crazy house whose apparent doors are mysteriously barred, whose entry points are impenetrable and whose views are without perspective or horizon.

With so many East London industries gone for good, there are few jobs which are reliable and through which orderly promotion is possible. Instead it's bits and pieces, ducking and diving, a fiddle here and a bit of self-exploitation there. Be a security guard until the contract is revised, work for the hospital until the next round of cuts, do a 'scheme'. Employment is nowadays chancy and arbitrary: likely to shut off at short notice, abolished when the next contractors are brought in. And family finances are permanently in a state of social insecurity.

When I started in East London, it had not only steady jobs but unions and apprenticeships. Now, famous acronyms like AEU, UCATT, NASD, are as dead as the docks themselves. Yet, after the decade-long assault on trade unionism, welfare and public housing, little, apart from the very mixed blessings of the LDDC, was gained. The work the patients do is still mainly manual, associated with distribution, catering and petty manufacture, with a lot of women in low-paid, low-prestige, high-demand work in the NHS and the education services: the receptionists, secretaries, clerks and cleaning ladies who keep the services from collapse. Those who still work for the once great public services – for the Post Office, or the Gas Board, or as train and bus drivers – are increasingly fed-up with privatisation and petty managerialism, cynical and embittered about the next gimmick, angry at the growing differentials between those who do and those who administer. And all find the working environment of late twentieth-century London harsher, harder and more ungrateful. Those out of work, although more effectively harassed to retrain, are still failing to get work, not because of lack of motivation but because of the mismatch between the results and skills their traditional East End education has equipped them with and the demands of the new jobs coming out of the City of London.

As for income, the statistics tell us that more inner city dwellers are entering the band of subsistence. And this is exacerbated in the East End by the poll tax which hits large families where several generations commonly live in a single household especially hard. But statistics are hard to flesh, especially because we tend to see our imagery of poverty in terms of the previous generation's suffering and miss what is under our own noses. Cars, if owned at all, are old, beaten-up and require a great deal of owner maintenance. But a car is essential for certain journeys to be made at all. Otherwise a baby buggy has to be used as a haulage cart for supermarket shops and the launderette, as well as a means to immobilise otherwise active children while queuing for doctor, dole, or giro. Clothes are not replaced till they are worn through and then are bought in markets, at sales, or from cheap mass retailers. Shoes, like teeth a telling indicator of income, are now trainers which are not watertight or warm and, even though East London was once an international centre of shoe- and boot-making, poorly made and ill-fitting imports. There was a time when an East End working man, however poor, would possess two respectable suits, a warm overcoat, a hat and a pair of leather boots. But the casualisation of male clothes conceals their impoverishment: men work on building sites, drink in pubs and take out their kids on Sunday in the same track suit and trainers. The East End tradition of knowing how to dress up for an outing has gone for a burton.

Food, its freshness, variety and quality, depends a great deal on shops. And there is no doubt that working-class nutritional standards were significantly improved by first tinned and then frozen goods. However, the dominance of supermarkets has made local food stores fewer and more expensive. And bread shops which had bakeries in the rear are now rare, a single chain controlling most of the East End bread and cake trade. I can remember having bakers as patients, big round men usually with arthritis of the hands, who would tell of the days when the servants in the big houses would sell off their surplus baking to neighbours from the basement window. And fish, which with oyster and shellfish was a staple of the nineteenth-century East End diet, is hard to buy, except in its mutilated form as fish fingers, despite the presence in the borough of Billingsgate, the specialist fish market.

So, while the middle classes become more food- and health-conscious and take steps to modify the traditional British diet so rich in fat and red meats, in East London traditional food marches on. Pies and sausages, oven-ready chips and other convenience foods load up the shopping trolleys in Asda and Tesco; chips and milkshakes are eaten out and breakfast is a cigarette and a cup of instant coffee. Cigarette-smoking is actually increasing, a lethal habit acquired by new immigrants from Vietnam and Bangladesh and popular with school-children, girls as much as boys. This tradition, like heavy beer- and spirits-drinking, may be related to the docks and the subsidised cigarettes which sailors brought ashore. Some patients insist it was the Blitz and wartime factory work which started them smoking.

Much current concern about diet assumes that the problem is only of people eating too much, especially too much animal fat. This type of obesity is very common in East London, causing much morbidity. But I see a good deal of old-fashioned low-intake malnutrition, especially among the old and the long-term unemployed; people who will survive on sweet tea, toast, chips and biscuits. Bread and margarine is a dietary staple in the 1990s as much as it was in the 1930s. Pregnant women and children under five are commonly found to be anaemic and the elderly and the physically handicapped are often made more vulnerable to illness by the inadequate quantity of the food they can afford. Women commonly cut back on their own food to feed their children and husband. Food is often short by the end of the week. In large families it often lacks variety, freshness and quantity.

The credit boom of the 1980s has meant that debt is larger than ever before for all income groups. The Thatcher era's costly encouragement of home ownership had clear political intentions, like the widening of share ownership; it was aimed to provide a material incentive for working- and lower-middle-class voters to break with Labour. The source of home ownership has been council homes peeled off the local authority regardless of the damage done to the local economy and the housing market. And many of those people who stampeded into getting a mortgage at the height of the hard sell were by the 1990s repenting at leisure as the mortgage rate skipped from 9 per cent to 15 per cent; we are a mortgage-paying rather than property-owning democracy. A 1990 Policy Studies Institute report on debt found one in nine of British families in serious arrears, with the problem worst in families with a weekly income of under £100. The commonest indebtedness was council rent arrears. Although the well-off had increased their borrowings, they had the flexibility to manage their debt. But poorer creditors who often don't qualify for charge cards or HP agreements, had to pay higher interest for their borrowings from loans and credit sharks. Frequently, poorer East End families owe money to several companies and start paying one off only to switch their efforts when the debt collector from the next puts on the pressure. So young families are often juggling gas and electricity bills, overdrafts, store-card invoices and the rent. They then borrow high-interest cash loans to attempt to clear the deck and dig themselves into a still bigger hole. The problem, insufficient income, doesn't go away. Most single parents and unemployed families have some outstanding debt, and about 15 per cent of patients have three or more arrears. It is this unforgiving pressure, rather than propensity to sin, which is at the back of the pathetically petty crime which the East End papers list each week, and which has caused the return of street prostitution to the East End, no longer confined to the traditional 'red light' areas of Whitechapel but under the bridges in Bethnal Green, down the back streets of Stoke Newington and in Hackney pubs . . . 'Thatcher's girls', the locals call them. People shoplift not out of greed or laziness but sheer need: the giro stops and the baby's hungry. Yet, if caught, the mother can end up in prison for it. Sometimes the stories told by patients don't seem so very far from the nineteenth century after all.

Poverty rose especially sharply in the East End because of the exceptionally high levels of real unemployment, between 20 and 25 per cent throughout the decade. But by 1985, 9.4 million people in the UK, including 2.25 million children, were living at or below the official poverty line. This is 17 per cent of the population – an increase of 55 per cent since 1979. The number of children in poverty nearly doubled. Two-thirds of disabled people, about 4 million, live at or below the poverty line. But in Tower Hamlets, the most proletarian of the London boroughs, with such a high proportion of unskilled manual labourers, as many as a third of the patients are below the formal poverty line and another third are at its margins. Talk of boom-time Britain and the opportunity society is an ugly joke to the poorest tenth of society whose average real income, after allowing for housing costs, increased between 1979 and 1987 by a negligible 0.1 per cent as compared to the average rise of 23 per cent and the stupendous rise in wealth of the top 2 per cent who already own more than the bottom 75 per cent put together. Teenagers under the age of eighteen were effectively excluded from benefit they had previously been able to obtain. Loans from the 'Social Fund' replaced cash payments for items urgently needed. No wonder more teenage runaways (more notified to the Limehouse police district than in the whole of the remainder of North-East Thames – over 500 in 1990 including 56 under twelve) end up in crime, drug-dealing, prostitution, or, quite often, all three. And no surprise that many of the loan requests to the Social Fund, for such things as rubber sheeting for the inconti-nent, cookers, overcoats and bar fires, are refused because their commitments are already too extensive to guarantee that they will be able to make the repayments – in other words, because they are too poor.

Poverty has been shown to cause ill-health by a grow-ing body of detailed medical research work over the last decade. There are very marked differences in the outcome of pregnancy according to social class, includ-ing late miscarriages, stillbirths and congenital deform-ities. Although infant mortality in all classes has improved, the improvement remains very relative: women of social class 5 (over 70 per cent of the East End population) have only now achieved outcomes enjoyed by women of social class 1 in the 1930s. Between the age of one and four years, the class gradi-ent remains very pronounced. Since the principal causes of death are from respiratory disease, accidents and neoplasm, such class-related factors as the degree of domestic overcrowding, the availability of safe public playspace, car ownership, access to good-quality medical care and the levels of pollution and nutrition are determining factors. These trends are clearly long-term: if a more equitable redistribution of wealth were to take place tomorrow, its medical consequences would not show till the next century.

The physical environment of the East End varies wildly; patches of great beauty and solitude are next to overflowing land-tip sites where toxins are lain in shallow graves, tangles of car bodies rust among heaps of newspaper, bottles and cans, canals bubble with bleach, rats and industrial effluent. There are semi-permanent traffic jams, foul air, dirty trains, filthy streets, vandalised litter bins. It is tough, decaying and depressing to grow up in.

Homelessness, which is the most extreme form of poverty, has doubled during the 1980s, with a quarter of a million homeless officially but probably more than that if childless couples and vagrants were properly included. According to the Joseph Rowntree Trust, the number of homeless families is increasing by 14 per cent per year. Here the full medical and psychological consequences of poverty are seen, and the difficulties individuals have attempting to break out of the downward spiral of deprivation however hard they try. East London had several large boarding houses built for the temporary housing of seamen, and these have now either been taken over by charities or private landlords, or converted to flats by housing associations. Thus in Limehouse, the British Sailors' Society is now private flats; the handsome Queen Anne Swedish Seamen's Mission in Garford Street, founded by the eccentric Baroness Leijonhjelm, is now a 500-bed Salvation Army hostel; and the Empire Memorial Sailors' Hostel, a gaunt building at the corner of Salmon Lane, was reopened as the notorious Princes Lodge. This Piranesi-like maze of corridors and narrow partitioned-off bedrooms, privately owned, was used for local homeless families, especially pregnant single mothers awaiting council accommodation, but was also occupied by young people coming to London in search of work and homeless Bangladeshi families. These hostels developed as a private and very profitable response to the housing crisis, rent being paid directly through Social Services. The hostels were not suitable for children or for long-term accommodation, although the homeless often stay there for over a year. The buildings are often fire traps and frequently overcrowded. In Princes Lodge there were no proper facilities for cooking or food storage; people lived off takeaways and lager. If food was stored, especially in summer, it went off, got infested, or was stolen. In the midst of this squalor, young families did their best to construct a zone of decency. Husbands would go out for casual cash-in-hand work or spend hours on the phone to the housing department where, if they got through, the person handling their case would be out or 'in a meeting'. The same sink had to be used for cleaning nappies as well as mixing baby's feeding bottles. The children were often delayed in development, understimulated, prone to infection, skin problems, or bedwetting, their mothers exhausted but sleepless, depressed but chattering to keep their spirits up. So many of their problems related to housing that the health visitors were obliged to become honorary housing workers.

Of those officially homeless in Tower Hamlets there were, on 1 April 1989, 1,098 families in temporary accommodation, an estimated 6,000 people, the majority of whom were housed outside the borough. This is over ten times as many as the national average. Although there has been increased use of short-life, hard-to-let council properties within the borough, like John Scurr House for emergency housing for the homeless, the position is worsening, for a number of reasons. Right-to-buy schemes and privatisation of estates by the Liberal local authority is taking the newest and most attractive homes out of the housing stock. Private housing prices, even so-called 'affordable' ones, are way above what a low-income family can consider. There is little private renting existing or likely to become available, and both new council building and renovation are severely limited by government financial legislation. Tower Hamlets places families into bed-and-breakfast while it examines their case. If 'unintentionally' homeless, they are transferred to private licensed accommodation. If not, they are served with an eviction order; so waiting is exceptionally stressful.

The full scale of the housing crisis is far larger than the poor souls sleeping rough in the sheds and skips and gutters of the East End or the families in B-and-B. It is now impossible for a qualified and full-time employed married couple in London, say a primary schoolteacher and a nurse whose weekly take-home pay in 1989 would be a total of £344, to afford a maximum mortgage of more than £47,000. Yet the average price of a one-bedroom home for first-time buyers in London was £63,700. Rented accommodation for the same couple would cost £125, and since they would not be eligible for Housing Benefit such a rent would take up 36 per cent of their combined income. They would stand absolutely no chance of eligibility for council housing; and housing association accommodation, the centrepiece of government policy but in fact a reversion to the late nineteenth century, is still small, getting smaller, and often has closed waiting lists. So if the people who teach your children and care for you in hospital can't even afford a home, what chance does a single parent or an immigrant family stand? And what exactly are you supposed to do if you don't have security of tenure and are made to leave, if you get ill or unemployed and fall behind with the mortgage, if you have to leave your partner because he was violent? Suppose they close the hospital you were in or you've just been released from prison? Or the friends who were putting you up can't do it any more or there's no room left in your parents' home when you have a child? Or you do something as simple as growing up? You don't have to be a dosser to be homeless. Yet this ludicrous and cruel situation is not the consequence of some natural calamity or war but the deliberate result of central government policy, which between 1981 and 1989 cut the number of houses let to new tenants by London councils by 41 per cent and the number of new council houses built by 91 per cent. During the same period, again as a deliberate policy, over 17 per cent of London council houses were sold off, further cutting the housing stock by 150,000 homes. It's not very surprising that the B-and-B business flourished, rising from an annual payment to hotel landlords of £4 million in 1981 to £99 million by 1987. What is genuinely shocking is that, as an act of policy, over £223 million has been handed by the ratepayers to the hotel landlords without the gain of a single unit of permanent housing for the homeless and at the cost of such cruel damage to the lives of so many adults and children. It is a policy which has generated its own momentum and will require great determination to reverse. In London, at the end of 1990, the local authorities estimate that another 4,000 families will go into B-and-B over the next eighteen months, making a total of 12,000 families.

It's not easy to forget the depression and the desperation of those hellish hotels; kiddies visibly failing to thrive and apathetic, parents glazed and ratty, the crumpled discharge letters from labour wards the other side of London, the lost baby books, the cockroaches and the endless, pointless housing letters. I still dream of Princes Lodge's ghastly corridors, lit like an expressionist film set, visiting mothers trying to comfort their newborn while next door runaways swig their Special Brew and methadone. I still can smell the over-sweet odour of Dettol, nicotine and rice pudding which pervades the sitting rooms of the Salvation Army hostel at Garford Street. And still dread the gentile shabbiness of Providence Row night shelter with its metal priest's hole for the homeless to beg the Sisters of Mercy for admittance at evening opening time and the neatly folded piles of clothes, one topped with a proud British Rail porter's cap, beside the camp beds. And every night about 250 people sleeping rough in Tower Hamlets. The 1980s may have been a decade of shining opportunity for some, for me it was the decade when one became hardened to the sight of hunched and dishevelled human bundles in doorways, disused buildings, even skips. Some enterprise, some culture.

The impact of prolonged high levels of unemployment goes even deeper than the poverty and homelessness. It creates a sense of despondency, worthlessness and eventually physical ill-health in individuals and despair in communities. Although some East London unemployment reflects the frictional (between-jobs) unemployment of a service economy catering to the City's need for cleaners, messengers, tea ladies and security guards, the majority of unemployed men are experiencing the structural change of the post-docks era. Thus a lock-keeper, made redundant when a private development firm took over the stretch of water he had worked for decades, applies energetically and optimistically for new jobs for three months and doesn't get an interview, then reapplies for his own job and sees an inexperienced younger man get appointed. And after six months out of work, he's a shadow of himself, having been divested not just of his working identity but his sense of worth, now getting anxiety attacks and angina which didn't trouble him when at work. Thus, too, a beefeater turned janitor, redundant docker, ex-printer, former lorry driver: one comes to recognise a loss of hope in their faces and in the familiar complaints of insomnia, dyspepsia, chest and back pain and depression.

The social cost of chronic unemployment is even more severe. In the 1930s, Marie Jahoda carried out pioneering sociological studies on the Austrian village of Marienthal in the period between the closure of the single large factory which dominated employment and

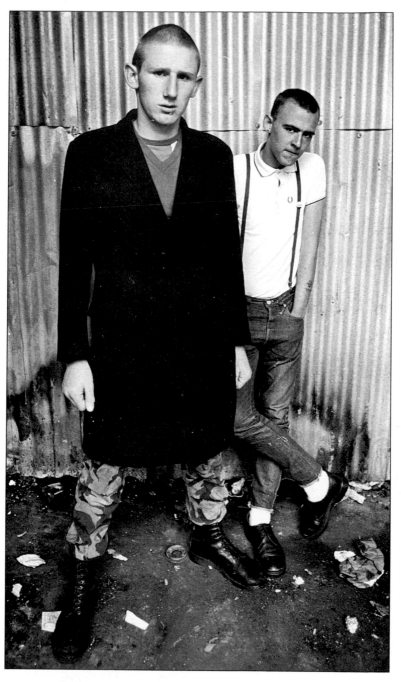

Part of the National Front Squadron which attempted a
Kristallnacht in Brick Lane on 11th June 1978.

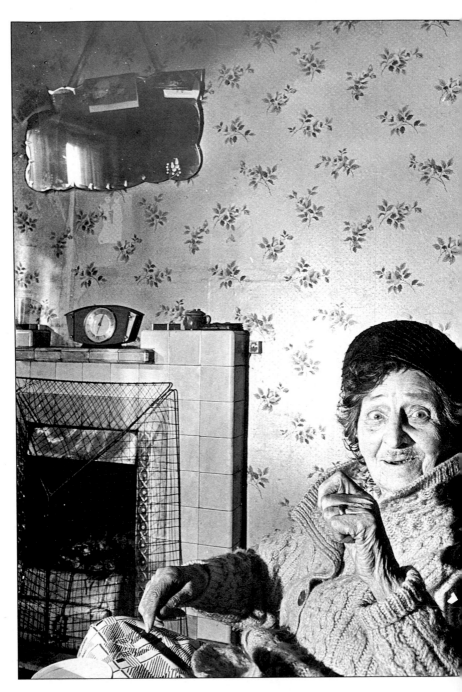

Old, alone and cold in Bow ... admitted to hospital with pneumonia
hypothermia.

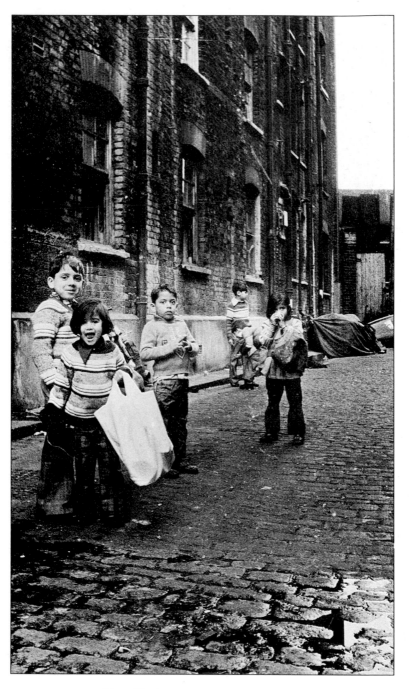

East End street urchins ... 1990.

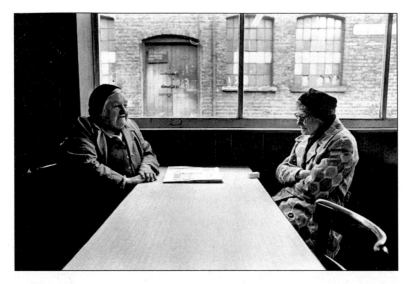

A proletarian breakfast in the Sandwich Bar opposite Dr Leibson's
Bethnal Green Road surgery.

Diabetic complications in Bow;
patient has lost her sight and both legs.

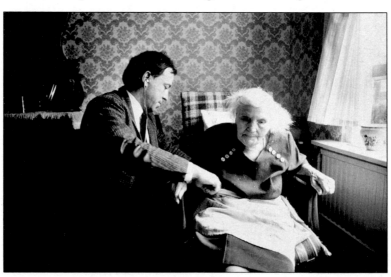

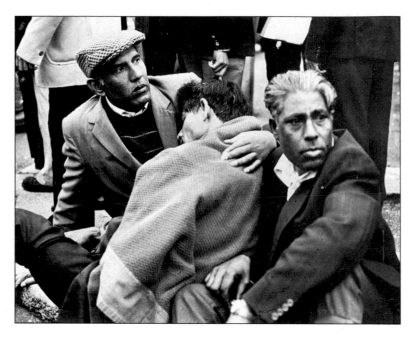

Asian brewery workers ambushed and pelted with rocks in
Three Mills Lane, Bow on 6th July 1978.

Saul, the furrier in Bethnal Green:
'he gets a few drinks and wants to wipe everyone out'.

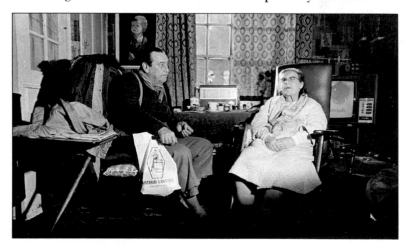

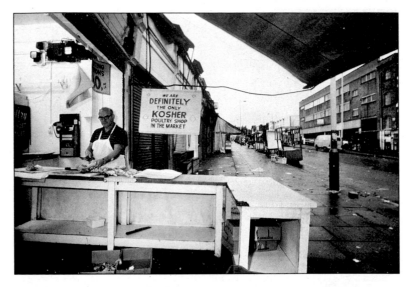

Ridley Road Street Market at dawn: the vestiges of old Orthodoxy.

On Sunday evening call out St Vincent's Estate, Limehouse ...
recently mugged.

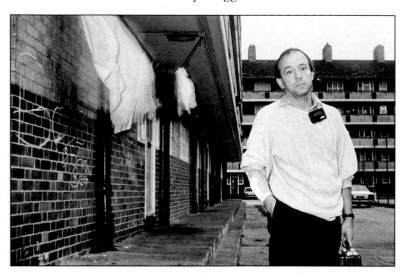

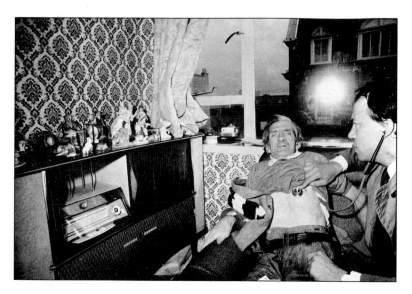

Pulmonary tuberculosis above the
Roman Road Street Market, Bow.

Bangladeshi Cockneys: sisters in Limehouse.

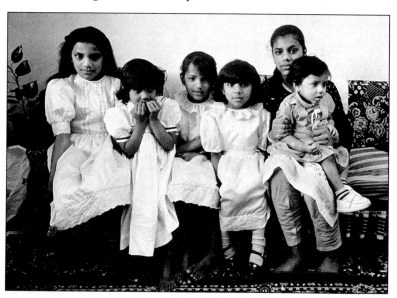

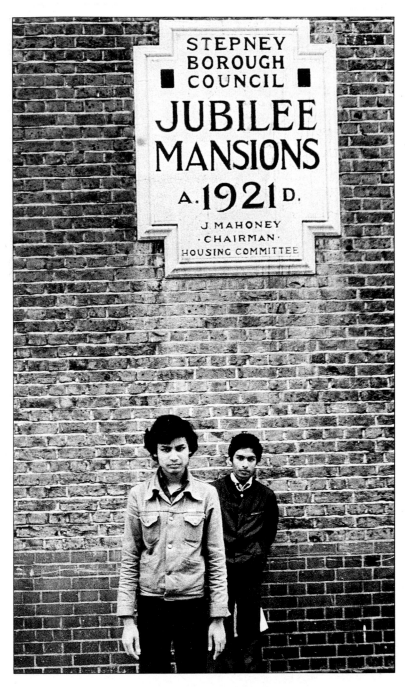

Asian youths outside improved dwellings built in Stepney by one of London's first Labour Councils.

the arrival of Hitler with soup kitchens, warm uniforms and conscription. Her group's account is grim and familiar reading in three ways. First, it demonstrates that the loss of self-esteem precipitated by loss of work cannot easily be remedied by attempts to compensate for lost earnings by unemployment benefit, free newspaper subs, or reduced-price entrance fees. Second, it reminds us that the mass unemployment of the Great Depression was 'solved' only by the Second World War, and that the long postwar boom was also underpinned by the Cold War arms economies of Washington and Moscow. Our post-Cold War market economies are also high-unemployment economies – they are bound to be if the market in the East, the West and the Third World is to operate untrammelled. Far from having eliminated the human, medical and social waste of mass unemployment, we are likely to witness its rapid expansion, notably to Eastern Europe and the Soviet Union where the decades of Stalinism incubated rather than eliminated the toxins of anti-Semitism and fascism. Thirdly, she notes the profoundly demoralising effect the absence of fruitful work is to the body politic as well as to the individual physiognomy. Work imposes a time structure on the waking day; it enlarges the scope of social relations beyond the family and the immediate neighbourhood; by virtue of the division of labour it demonstrates that the purposes and achievements of a collectivity transcend those for which an individual can aim. It gives life traction, it teaches regularity, it gets you out of bed in the morning. It also, in East London, has offered men and women the experience, through trade unionism, of collective strength and solidarity. We sneer at the crudity of the old 1930s slogans like 'Unemployment leads to fascism and war' at our peril. For prolonged unemployment does have politically corrosive results, it breeds resentment and frustration which can all too easily be channelled into racialism, xenophobia and chauvinism. Jahoda wrote in the 1930s: 'We entered Marienthal as scientists; we leave

121

with only one desire: that the tragic opportunity for such an inquiry may not recur in our time.' Her desire was not fulfilled.

Once out of work and unsuccessful in interviews, on the receiving end of embarrassed condescension and thank you, no, thank you, a fatalism which adapts to a lesser form of life is quickly adopted. This is often made bearable with alcohol for the older and drugs for the youngsters. Booze, even if swigged in a bus shelter or grim back bar, has some collective conviviality. And the business of getting, selling and consuming illicit drugs almost replaces some of the functions of a job. For in the modern world, with the traditional working-class unions, clubs and institutions eroded, the unemployed are more adrift, more alone and their personal resources more cruelly mocked by the TV world of compulsive consumption. Unemployed people just don't try out interesting recipes with pulses and natural yogurt; in their kitchenette lie a bag of sugar, a plastic box of margarine and a sliced white loaf. Unemployed people, on the whole, don't use spare time to organise anti-poll tax committees or unemployed workshops: they sit glumly staring at TV, smoking Silk Cut. And the young, who have never experienced the rewards of work, are even more deadened by its loss. The philosophy of 'why bother?' takes over.

Something as simple as a free bus pass, a successful grant application, even a friendly reception at the doctor's surgery, can be of importance in halting this lethal decline of morale. And encouragement for a job, however lousy, and then joining a union or an anti-cuts committee means a lot. I often write references for patients, and it's striking how narrow the employment options become for a male skilled industrial worker once out of work for more than six months. They tramp London to apply for basic warehouse and catering jobs, and when there is a hospital portering or post office vacancy the competition is fierce. On the 'No Entry' signs at the local building sites is scrawled, with-

out exception, the handwritten addition 'No Jobs'.
Unemployment means more consultation with the GP,
often for hypochondriacal illness, which used to be
known as 'neurasthenia', sometimes quite dramatic,
often difficult to diagnose safely without some investigation.

·Unemployed people, most noticeably young single
mothers, also lose, or never acquire, confidence in dealing with health matters. They are more likely to consult
doctors for minor complaints which they are perfectly
capable of dealing with themselves. And there is now
very well documented evidence of the raised incidence
of mental illness, especially depression and suicide,
among the unemployed (suicide remains a significant
cause of male premature death in the East End). And
despite the technical difficulties and lack of government
interest in financing research, there is now impressive
evidence of a positive association between unemployment and physical pathologies. As the NHS in East
London, despite the valiant efforts of those who work
in it, remorselessly declines, the number of those need-
ing its help seems set to grow.

CHAPTER 8

---∘◉∘---

NOT GOING GENTLY

Social change in the twentieth century, within which medical science played only a minor part, has extended the expectancy of life for all classes. At the turn of the century, it was unusual to live to three score years and ten. The poignant epitaphs in the older East End graveyards at Abney Park and Mile End show why. Death in childhood was commonplace and many adults perished in their thirties and forties. Infectious illness was the principal cause of mortality and, before the antibiotic era, GPs had a largely ceremonial and comforting role since they were unable to materially alter the course of illness. But by the end of the century, the proportion of old and very old (seventy-five years or more) in the population has increased, in East London, to about one in six. And this is low compared with the coastal retirement areas and depopulated rural Britain: the East End's high levels of immigration keep its population artificially young. Not only do people live longer but, in general, the birth rate has fallen.

For the elderly, their own financial assets and their level of family support are the two most important determinants of well-being. The affluent elderly *are* in the prime of their life. Exactly as pictured in the pension adverts, they are enjoying the fruits of their lives, relishing the challenge of their gardens and the company of their grandchildren. But for the East End pensioner, the picture is often the reverse: poverty and isolation. The present generation of the very old, say those born before the First World War, were typically members of big families but had few children themselves (the fertility rate dropped dramatically in the 1920s, largely due to the mass availability to working-class women of the means of reliable family planning). And those children, if they have got on, have got out of the East End. Even if they have remained, the arbitrary laws of the council-house allocation system mean they are unlikely to live nearby. A significant proportion of women will not have married or are widows. Not only will the immediate family members who can 'take care' be few and scattered, but the elderly will rely for income on the state pension. They will tend, out of pride or ignorance, not to take up the various means-tested income supplements. They will be council tenants who, unlike home owners, have not accumulated property assets and whose housing costs go up rather than down in later life.

Rather than old age being some universal state of being, it reflects quite precisely the class circumstances of the life that preceded it. We are born physiologically broadly equal, but by our sixties our bodies bear the evidence of occupation and social conditions. Our duration of life and cause of death will be the end products of the inequalities in the use made of our bodies. And for surprising numbers of male manual workers, retirement after a hard working life, which was as physically demanding in their fifties as their twenties, is followed by premature death from preventable causes, from a stroke, lung cancer, or a heart attack. Perhaps more tragically still, an East End working life will often be followed, not by well-earned retirement but a non-fatal stroke or early dementia (Alzheimer's Disease) which will render a once independent and active person chronically dependent. There can be few more devastating changes than the transformation which occurs when a stroke renders a previously articulate and agile partner speechless and chair-bound. Or when a wife of forty years deteriorates mentally so as to require constant supervision, incapable of anything but repetitive, incomprehending gibberish.

But to talk about the old as 'geriatric' is to see them immediately as ill and therefore dependent. Whereas many are, within the biological limits of the ageing process, active, alert and fiercely independent. It is to see them simply as an age category rather than individual people who deserve respect as mothers and lovers and storytellers and historians. For every person over sixty-five who has a home help, there are nine who don't. For everyone living in a local authority old people's home, there are fifty who don't.

Rather than 'suffering' from old age, East End pensioners are done down by something very much simpler – lack of finances. And the principal cause of that poverty is a paltry state pension which rewards the generation who fought through both the Great Depression and the Blitz with a mean stipend which bears no relation to real wage levels. The retired workers who have lived thrifty lives but who have neither property nor investments are likely in their old age to be very poor by general standards. Poor means often cold and at risk of death during extreme winter weather. It means eating a very basic diet with little variety and often low in vitamins, on foil trays from the Meals on Wheels during the day and out of tins at night and weekends. It means shabby, well-worn clothing, purchased secondhand and infrequently cleaned. It means rarely a car and seldom a washing machine. It means a life spent indoors watching the TV to the end and hoping the knock on the door is not an intruder. One doesn't need any statistical equipment more complicated than a pair of eyes to observe this. Look, for example, at the foray at the knitted clothes stall at East End jumble sales and observe the broken boots and laddered stockings in any geriatric outpatients. Watch pensioner couples, perplexed by prices, putting too costly items back on to supermarket shelves. See the queue for sweet tea and free biscuits at the pensioners' clubs or the old gentlemen in the back of the public bar nursing their half pints hour by hour. Look into the eyes of a pensioner living alone (one in six of British households) and, by and large, you see not serenity and comfort but fear, impatience and the desire to be somewhere, anywhere, else.

Yet by 2001, the over-seventy-fives will have grown to 40 per cent of pensioners. And on present evidence their need for medical and social services will be considerable. Already patients aged seventy-five and older make up a third of all hospital patients, two-thirds of the disabled and almost three-quarters of the severely handicapped. They will be, or should be, high users of the NHS and statutory services. This is not, as is popularly conceived, because they are past it or worn out and need some sort of institutional storage prior to expiry. Rather, many have medical problems which, if correctly diagnosed and treated, can, with appropriate social support, prolong independence. Far from geriatric medicine being an intellectually less rigorous or rewarding field, it is increasingly one of great diagnostic sophistication. The differentiation between undiagnosed mental illness and confusion due to reversible physical causes, or the differential diagnosis of weight loss in the elderly, requires experience and skill: it's far too easy just to nod 'anno domini' wisely and leave relatives to get on with it. And dementia itself, a scourge whose scale is still unacknowledged, may well be eventually more accurately subdivided into clinical entities which will probably include some that are amenable to active treatment.

It is often because of lack of financial resources and social isolation that people need Meals on Wheels and home helps: if they had microwaves and could afford home grocery deliveries, they would probably prefer to do it themselves. And if they could motor to a

127

country hotel, they would prefer that to the council's biannual trip to Clapton, now cut. Working-class pensioners aren't different, in their desire for independence, from younger adults. They haven't mysteriously transmogrified into a species of overgrown enfeebled children. Rather, their wages during a life of manual work will have tended to decline in their last decades rather than increase annually. They will therefore have been less likely to afford an occupational pension or to have acquired long-term financial assets. And the real value of their pension represents a dramatic fall in standard of living and thus expectations. East End pensioners are not incapable of enjoying cruise ships or banquets, they are just too busy saving up for their bus pass.

But quite aside from the question of a just pension that is related automatically to the national average wage, the rise in the number of old people will inevitably need a great expansion of all services, from long-term hospital beds, through old people's homes and sheltered warden-controlled flats, to subsidised telephones, cheap travel and home adaptations. Instead, these public services have been starved of funds. And spending per patient on the elderly in the NHS is less than average, suggesting a less good service. The unspoken attitude is that the elderly, because closer to death, merit only second-division care. In 1982 the House of Commons Select Committee on Social Services predicted: 'There is widespread recognition that the care of the frail elderly represents the major challenge in personal social services over the decades ahead. . . . That we should be already falling behind cannot but be disturbing and bodes ill for services to the elderly in future years.' Since then things have got progressively worse. And the handing over to local authorities of responsibility for the bulk of the care of the elderly, although administratively logical, is bound to worsen underfunding, especially in the East End where poll tax set at levels which are realistic will be unable to meet the likely costs. Instead the pattern of uneven quality of services, arbitrarily assigned and incoherently administered, is likely to persist and intensify.

The consequences of this remorseless problem are largely invisible. This is not just because the decline in the condition of the home-bound takes place out of public sight, but because many of the statutory services which are cut or simply were never available are provided 'free', but at great personal cost to those concerned, by 'carers', also invisible. Picture an outrageously demented old lady suffering from dementia. She is not simply withdrawn and mildly confused. Instead she rushes disinhibited at the walls shouting and swearing in bouts and then breaking into sobbing floods of tears. Her swearing is neither conversational nor discreet: instead she strings together like beads the dirtiest words she has heard. This discomforts her distracted husband more than anything. 'She was such a lady,' he murmurs apologetically, 'once.' The rooms are bare except for a few phone numbers written in large letters; it looks unloved and stark, like a public cloakroom. All the little pieces of furniture and detail which make a room's identity have gone: she periodically hurls them at the wall. A home help, paid for privately by a relative, 'pops in'.

What is sobering about this demented situation, which would seem intolerable to anyone visiting for the first time, is that it has a kind of equilibrium. The husband still loves his wife, recognises the bride he married through this scatological diatribe, wants to care for her at home. She is too densely demented for the community psychiatric nurses, who *can* do wonders for the anxious and the lonely, to make any impact. She refuses to leave the house to visit a day centre, and pills either don't get taken or make no impact on her furious rages and stormy tears. She needs a permanent psychogeriatric bed, indefinite section to a secure ward of a mental hospital. But there are only 5 of these for a population of 166,000. And anyway, her husband would refuse to sign the papers. In a curious way, if he can take it, she's better off at home.

Likewise the wife of an ex-lorry driver who has a part-time City job as a messenger. She first complains he's unresponsive and aggressive in the evening and there are dreadful arguments over the TV. It could be marital, it could be lunchtime drinking, she could be neurotic. When he comes to surgery, he denies any problems and seems, on simple memory-testing to be OK. His blood tests are normal too. Then the son confirms something's wrong with Dad: he's putting the sliced bread in the oven and cutting up the lino; then staying out late and unable to say where he's been. It must be Alzheimer's, although he's only sixty-four and manages to conceal it well from me. But he contrives to be out when the psychogeriatrician calls and now refuses completely to come to the surgery. The family are getting desperate. The wife lies awake all night and cries herself to sleep when he's finally in bed: 'He's not the man I married,' she – accurately – cries. The son just thinks Dad's being a bastard: 'He always was.' Eventually the police take him, battered and bleeding, into custody on a Section 136. I see him next in the secure psychogeriatric ward where patients wander in worlds of their own behind locked doors. He doesn't recognise me, his wife, or his son any longer. Just stands miming sorting the post. He remains in the ward, in that state, for the next eighteen months until he dies quite rapidly of lung cancer. His wife visits once a week with little presents of cake and home-made pies which he gives away immediately to other patients. He never spoke her name again. 'And his language, Doc, it was shocking.'

Immense strain was put on the carers which had consequences long, long after their spouses eventually gained admission to scarce institutional care. Alfred, whose scatological wife was eventually admitted under Emergency Section at night when he finally broke an arm and *had* to go to hospital, misses her terribly.

Unwilling to visit, he has become depressed himself and reclusive. The bank messenger's wife, now bereaved, can't get transferred from the house they shared together and in which he went demented. She is still grieving for a partner whom she lost as a person two years before he died. It is that private grief and strain which is the cost of the withdrawal of public services. But it doesn't enter on the profit or loss sheets and so is never calculated. No bed is closed. But if it had a human price on it, it would be a high one.

Most elderly people, even with chronic illness, manage well with minimum medical intervention. But when care isn't tailored properly, or simply because of a sequence of accidents, a crisis can blow up. Someone wrongly allowed sleeping tablets by repeat prescription may wake early in the morning and, still intoxicated by their medication, trip and break a brittle hip. They are admitted by a 999 call to an orthopaedic bed. They survive the fall and the surgery but might then die or become disorientated as a consequence of admission. Too often elderly patients admitted to hospital during a bout of acute illness are discharged abruptly without proper arrangements being made, and then flounder badly, quite often requiring readmission. This is not a matter of attitude: all doctors and nurses understand the importance of making planned discharge arrangements, especially for the elderly. Rather it's the failure of good intentions when engulfed with the sheer work load. So it is that old people, seen demeaningly as potential 'bed blockers', are turfed out on Fridays, either to make bed space for the next wave of emergencies, or because the hospital is economising on weekend staff.

So when things aren't arranged right, someone recovering from an illness but not yet fully fit might land up without the services that had previously kept them functioning. There are no Meals on Wheels, the home help isn't reinstated and the family are left to dish out the new pills without the help of the district nurse. Convalescence, so beloved of our medical predecessors, has gone with the Cuts. So old people are put back into the very conditions, including damp housing and poor diet, which have contributed to their admission, to await the next crisis. At its worst it can end with a battle of wits between a chronically ill patient who wants to be admitted and a hospital and GP team who are trying to bolt together adequate community services. This becomes still more problematic when the patient is also demented, depressed, or confused. A casualty officer, who effectively guards the entry portals to the hospital's scarce beds, will patch up the bruises, stitch the wounds and send home if possible. In the brave new world of health service reform, it will be impossible to admit patients on 'social' grounds . . . that's somebody else's problem. So casualty officers are increasingly put in the position of the old Poor Law officers; and admit less on grounds of medical logic but more on whether patients can be made to fit a clinical category (or, even worse, demonstrate a useful teaching sign). Others who can just about survive on their own are sent home, sometimes by minicab. As admission becomes increasingly pressured, GPs are called out, usually over the weekend, to become adjudicators in a family crisis. And often the elderly person is not the central figure at all but the relative or carer who 'just can't cope any longer'. The alleged invalid is often quite serene, but the daughter is sobbing quietly and the son-in-law who's motored in from Dagenham is full of moral ire: 'What are you going to do about it, Doctor?' What you tend to do about it is haul the old lady upstairs or get her to do whatever else was the sticking point and promise a respite admission A.S.A.P. But these respite admissions, a planned break for the carers, are only a token, no substitute for the more intensive material support which should be available to the, usually female, relatives who have had to become full-time home nurses.

Caring becomes more difficult as death approaches. Death is the great truth of all our lives; however sharp-witted, fit, or rich, we can't avoid it, and yet, in the modern world, we are unlikely to have experienced it at home. When people want their dying to be put in hospitals, it is only partly because they hope for treatment which will save them. In reality it is because we can't face death. It's everywhere in fiction: it is said a Californian child will have seen 2,000 deaths on TV by the time it's five. But we know nothing of it firsthand, how unappeasable and cruel it is, what it's like when it happens. Instead we tidy it away with 'floral tributes', funeral directors and the witless rhetoric of the crematorium dirge. For death, for most working-class patients, isn't usually kind or 'a release' or all the other slippery phrases which lie about it. It's the final confirmation that many of life's possibilities have been confiscated. To take the pain and the injustice out of death is the meanest sentimentality. It is something starker: I have seen too often the gasping and fading in a room which has accumulated only the most meagre of possessions, the last struggle of a body that has known little luxury and much settling for less.

As a doctor, your next encounter is with a corpse which you are, for the purposes of cremation, required to examine in the rear of the undertaker's. The front lounges of these places are well upholstered, full of cigarette smoke and euphemisms, but the bodies are usually stored out of sight in a clanking garage-like morgue whose slightly putrid smell is not completely masked by detergent. The body is now cold, stiff and often toothless, in a galvanised container. Death makes people ugly. Ugly because inert; the sweat and lung-suck and heartbeat gone. Hard to believe this person has ever worked, thought, journeyed, fantasised, or procreated. Now a passenger at the rites, while taped organs intone and priest pontificates.

GPs are still required to 'certify' death, another ritual which is legal rather than medical. And this is a moment, and an important one, to meet relatives who are grieving. A family who have been nursing a ter-

minally ill patient at home sometimes need a formal
statement of death, a piece of paper to make it real.
What you say at this moment is important; even the
banal words of sympathy can mean a lot. At least East
Enders know how to mourn: they have to. Like the
old Irish and Jewish families, all ages sit with each
other and the body. Rooms fill with relatives you don't
know, sobbing, clutching and supporting each other,
streaming sons and tearful grandchildren assembled
instantaneously even at 4 a.m. You feel for the absent
pulse, shine a light into unresponsive pupils, shake endless hands and refuse sweet tea, swallowing instead a
bitter mixture of relief and sadness. A moment which
is very strong.

It is more painful to be called to a person who has
died unattended and alone. These are the bodies keeled
over in the toilet or stiff in a stale bedroom, blue and
contorted in the time they have lain undiscovered. Once
I was called to a flat where a man had become depressed,
drunk himself to death and sat for six days rotting on
top of a vast mound of empties, like a Guy Fawkes
consumed by drink instead of flames. The smell was
rich and sickly and he was almost impossible to reach
and examine on his pyre of debris. Unexpected death
is also frightening, although mostly the ambulance service is called before the GP and takes the body to the
hospital, often attempting revival even if it is clear the
person is dead. I remember trying to haul a stocky
butcher, who had died of a heart attack at 2 a.m. in
front of the TV, on to his bed, which seemed a better
resting place. But he doubled up as we lifted him and
the raised intra-abdominal pressure made it look as if
he took a breath. His widow insisted on mouth to
mouth again, and even though it was quite hopeless I
complied for a decent interval. 'Why did you take so
long?' is the question either spoken or unspoken when
one arrives at a deathbed. But it is rare that speed much
alters the course of events, although it is important for
those who are to live on to feel everything has been

134

done that could have been. As Epicurus says, death is no misfortune for him who died but for those who survived.

But how death is observed, the respect or otherwise human bodies are afforded, surely marks a measure of our degree of civilisation. In one week the local paper reported four East End deaths which were last exits of horror and neglect. A hospital porter in his fifties lay in a filthy local pond because 'the locals thought it was a bag of rubbish'. A Stepney pensioner was found dead only after a neighbour complained of a smell coming from his door. A Poplar widower hanged himself with a tie and a Hoxton man died alone of hypothermia after falling in his bedroom. Earlier in 1990, a ninety-one-year-old demented man lay dead in the grounds of Hackney Hospital for three weeks before discovery. A sixty-seven-year-old Clapton man drowned in a pool of roadside water that had developed when sewers had become blocked with mud and litter. During the 1989 flu epidemic, some of the Borough of Hackney's old people's homes were reported as being damp and draughty with a shortage of towels and sheets, intermittent hot water, dirty toilets and uncarpeted floors.

What is then bewildering is that such time, money and emotion are spent on the outward show of grief when it is all too late. But so little is done about the care of the old when they are living. What do we all want but a gentle death, near to those we have loved, with some sense that we have done some of what was possible and changed things for the better? To die peacefully *is* our greatest desire; to have 'come to terms' with death and no longer be petrified by the advance of 'the cure of all diseases'. To die fighting death is to cause yourself intractable pain. And I can remember people who have willed themselves to stay alive and the agony their demise has therefore become. A policeman with lung cancer who silently quaked with fury at the injustice of his illness. His family kept denying his death was a possibility and in futile solidarity pretended business as usual while he became skin and bones before their eyes. Yet other people can derive an almost exhilarating sense of purpose from the same situation and, instead of desperate anguish, derive great focus and intensity.

Like Mr Foley. Although a docker, Mr Foley had always been a little man. He was devoted to his rosy-cheeked, smiling, neatly made-up, welcoming wife. Their flat was in apple-pie order and he always attended on time for his blood pressure checks. Except one day when she, apologetically, called to cancel his appointment and ask me to visit myself. 'He's poorly today,' she said with a special tone. He was. Somehow exuding a new weakness, and welcoming me with an expression I had never seen on his kindly face before: a slight, beseeching look, half gratitude, half fear. I made to examine him with much jocular opening of my medical bag and reassuring brandishing of the stethoscope to give myself time to observe him. He had suddenly become bird-like: wrists tiny, cheekbones hollowed out, skin translucent. He had always been petit but now, only six weeks after I had last seen him, he had begun to be emaciated.

The shortness of breath was harder to evaluate: it can have so many causes. Except that his right upper chest sounds were very different in character and then, as he further undressed, I saw the give-away. On the skin of his left forearm was a hard knobbly growth, quite small but utterly distinct: a secondary skin cancer. Now flat on the sofa, I felt his abdomen gently. The liver was hard and distended and his ankles and feet were softly swollen with a dense, doughy oedema. Ca lung with skin secondaries, said my diagnostic forebrain: what a pity, what a pity, what can I say, recoiled my emotions. Looking his wife straight in the eyes, I strove not to falter. 'I think your husband had better go into the hospital this time. I'll arrange it straightaway.' And striving to be honest, I turned back to Mr Foley. 'We'd better find out what it's all about.'

Only two weeks later he died. At home. Sooner than I or anyone had expected. The district nurses were marvellous, finding sheepskins for his bedsore and book rests and high-calorie drinks. In that short time, I got to know Mr Foley as I had never done before: learnt about his singing down at the club, dressing up at parties, his sense of humour, the family's pride in the Foley brothers' record for staunch trade unionism in the Docks. I met his children and their in-laws, made attempts at consoling conversation and watched Arthur smile knowingly in his morphine-drowse. He died when his exhausted wife had just taken a nap for which she couldn't forgive herself. His tough son's face disintegrated when he recalled the moment. I saw him finally in the undertaker's, his face haggard but pristine, at peace, like a brass rubbing. Proud of his going.

It would be nice to think we were just departing to a congenial reunion of all those others we have loved who have died, waiting to welcome us to Hotel Eternity. Nice but implausible. What does linger is something almost more powerful, which is memory. It is the world which is given to us, as Cicero states, 'as an inn in which to stay, but not to dwell'. It is what we have done in life that lives on, not the trumped-up version of eternity which is worshipped in dank cemeteries and gravestone jingles. What we deserve to remember is real courage, not bogus virtue lauded at the funerals. How few deaths are 'acceptable': I was angry and hurt even when a ninety-six-year-old friend died. Indeed you can get lost in a pit of grief, determining you will never laugh or dance or joke again. But humans are enormously adaptable, have ways of healing their mental as well as physical pain. It's not the passage of time that matters, however, but what you do with it. Only with effort do we extract from the irreplaceable something that falls into place. The best description of this process I have found is in a letter of the 1870s by Marx's wife Jenny, herself ill with liver cancer, to the Sorges who had lost two children in the years of adolescence. She wrote:

> I know only too well how terrible it is and how long it lasts before one can again find one's equanimity in such a loss, but everyday life with its little pleasures and its great troubles, with all its petty worries and its minor torments, comes to our assistance and gradually the great suffering is numbed by the troubles and worries of the moment, so that almost unnoticeably the violent anguish diminishes; not that such wounds ever heal completely, and certainly not in a mother's heart, but gradually one recovers one's receptivity and even one's sensitiveness for new sufferings and new pleasures, and one lives on and on with a broken, but still hopeful heart.
>
> (Jenny Marx, 1878)

What is odd is that in our apparently highly sophisticated society, we are still cowardly about facing death. More incompetent and less civilised than the Greeks or even the Victorians. And that, even at the grave, there is such injustice. A great man's funeral is rich in decorum, music, honour and dignity. The pauper dies alone, floating like waste paper in a pond and puddle or rotting in the council flat.

CHAPTER 9

———◦❦◦———

GIN LANE/SKID ROW

The East End is London's traditional Skid Row. White-chapel in particular is a social sump into which the homeless, the severely mentally ill and the alcoholic are swirled. Nobody is quite sure why. In the case of schizophrenia (whose characteristic is *not* a 'split mind' but rather a delusional mental system and withdrawal from social life) which is a common illness affecting one in one hundred in all social classes, migration down the social scale is understandable. Sufferers are often rejected by their families and friends, lose work and therefore rapidly descend in social standing. So economic pressure, as well as the East End's greater tolerance of eccentric behaviour, brings them eastward as their illness worsens. Those with behaviour disturbances, especially related to violence, might also migrate because they can feel more at home in an area where physical aggression is more easily sanctioned. Alcoholics may also have been attracted by the availability of casual work and the willingness of some shopkeepers to sell meths and cheap lager to them at all hours. The pattern has been long established and the response to the pattern – the Salvation Army's main London hostels and drying-out centres are in Whitechapel and Limehouse, and there are other voluntary agencies with long histories in the area – attracts both new customers and professional referrals. What the mentally ill and the drink-dependent have in common is homelessness; the mainly male mobile population have often been thrown out of home, or never really had one, and have gravitated, via stretches in hostels, dry-outs and sleeping rough, across England to London and then across London to the East End.

The East End has a long tradition of heavy drinking. Waterside workers were often hired and paid in pubs (which in 1800 were said to account for one in seven of the buildings). And unsurprisingly, a good deal of these wages were spent at source. As in the mining areas, heavy manual work generated both a formidable thirst and the need for a quick-energy supply (alcohol is high in carbohydrates). As in the music hall songs, a wife was entitled to violence if her man didn't deliver his wages (or had drunk them). And rowdy weekend drinking, often with bawdy entertainment thrown in (at the penny gaffs) was traditional and legitimate; then as now, the uncanny quietness of the East End on Sunday morning is part of a collective hangover which stretches from Whitechapel to the Blackwall Tunnel. The East End was also, until very recently, the centre of the London brewing industry. Pubs are dense: one Bethnal Green street crossing had pubs on three of its four corners and, until the 1990 recession, Bethnal Green Road boasted seventeen. They are often rather grand and beautiful places representing a considerable investment by the brewers, flush with handsome returns. They uniquely combine fine architecture and interior fittings with a day-to-day utility; vernacular design if ever there was one. They also have kept alive the tradition of live variety entertainment and public political meetings which are so important to the East End.

The dockers were especially famed for their alcohol consumption; it was commonplace to set up a small bar on the job within the hold, supplied with filched grog, to restore spirits. And the dockside pubs, like the market bars, had special licences permitting them to serve drinks early in the morning. The momentum of the nineteenth-century temperance movement in East London therefore reflected not moral stinginess but the scale of excessive drinking. And the density of the charitable and missionary settlements in the East End, often in competition, marks the scale of the problem which was and is a frequent cause of domestic violence and family poverty.

The consequences of modern excessive drinking are not difficult to spot. Public intoxication is widespread and at all hours. The homeless drinkers sleeping rough in public parks, derelict sites and cardboard cities, often reserve a can or tot to get them started first thing, and are already buying the gleaming Special Brews or turquoise Tennants Super by breakfast-time. Any bohemian illusions about the romanticism of such a life should be weighed against the drinkers' faces and their physiques. The faces are simultaneously swollen and haggard, puffed with fluid retention and liver failure but drained by the malnutrition consequent on an alcohol-only dietary intake. Their eyes, bright remnants of a once vivid personality, are now just flickers in a dying fire. Their talk, the drunkard's delusion, is either pathetic imprecations, unsuccessful abuse, or manic jabber. It's hard to think these were once builders, carpenters, lab technicians, wheelwrights, publicans, lecturers. Yet their medical records, when you eventually track them down in a muddle of recent emergency medical admissions and unsuccessful dry-outs, start with an unremarkable early life as an industrial worker, a clerk, or a member of the armed forces.

In the Thatcher years, not only have their numbers grown in East London, but they are younger and more often mentally ill too. The worsening housing crisis and the closedown of the great asylums has increased public dementia and drunkenness and funnelled it into the East End. Their condition cannot be satisfactorily explained by an individual desire for self-destruction or original sin because their progress downhill has been a sequence of social events – loss of job, homelessness, poverty and imprisonment – which have interacted with the drinking. And, in a way, it is the women drinkers who are most desperate, their expressions either agonised or fake-merry, their ramshackle set of belongings hauled on a home-made cart, their drink often won by sexual barter or prostitution, yet kept away from the male drinkers' circle of bonhomie. Their state is less acceptable to a world which, deluded, sees the men's desperation as folkloric behaviour. They are tramps but she is a slag. Their lurching boasts are just an amplified version of the usual male pissed bravado but her begging is a disgrace against her sex. Their stringy locks are mock-heroic, her unwashed hair and akimbo lipstick a failed femininity.

I remember with special sadness an alcoholic woman – a tragic personal life but a good woman in many ways – whose drinking led her into prostitution and prevented her from taking proper radiotherapy for her breast cancer. I was often called to her tenement flat when her untreated carcinoma led to brain secondaries which caused her first to fall, then to fit. She medicated with a mixture of slow-release morphine, pills and Special Brew. Her common-law husband, pimp, or lover – depending on his mood and sobriety – sat playing dominoes with his friends in the smoke-filled sitting room. Although it was only 11 a.m., everyone was intoxicated. She said all she wanted me for was a certificate, but I bargained that I must examine her breast which was now fungating after its incomplete radiotherapy. There was hardly room for anything but a bed in the side room where she slept, and we both bounced on it while she undressed with a self-mocking coquettish air. But as she undressed, she slid into a grand mal fit and kicked the door, furiously flailing her arms and tongue. Unable to find a viable vein, I managed to get some diazepam in her buttock, and her boyfriend staggered off to phone an ambulance. She died that day without recovering consciousness.

Disinhibited, the drinkers are sometimes strangely kind; eager to talk to children, indiscriminately bonhomous. I remember seeing a drunken woman in the queue for the night shelter in Hanbury Street trying to cut a young man's shoulder-length hair and only succeeding in stabbing his cheek instead. But her incompetent act of human friendship seemed preferable to the two City types with squash bags who, literally, walked over them without pausing in their conversation. But as the day and the drink wears on, 'Man,' as Frans Masereel says, 'becomes a wolf to man'. There can be only momentary solidarity among the alcoholic lumpen. While conscious, the circle of scrubland cider drinkers may share a purpose, but as soon as one passes out or is spiked, another will settle an old score by kicking in his teeth. Tobacco is stolen off epileptics mid-fit, stiffs are robbed and even a friend is betrayed for a taste. The very ground around the park or graveyard is poisoned, dull and lifeless from years of being urinated on by winos. Women are as desperate and violent as men who, impotent through drink, despise them as whores sitting on a gold mine. Salvation is simply more money for drink, whether it comes through theft, robbery, or ingenious varieties of begging. It might end fittingly in self-devouring DTs in a TB-ridden, pill- and surgical-spirit-fuelled squat, or sleeping rough.

And even more dangerous than the incompetent internecine battles within the circle, are the attackers for whom the vagrant is fair game. For also roaming the city of dreadful night are people whose disturbed state is manifest not in the inward self-destruction of the chronic alcoholic but by aggressive and violent external behaviour. The classic skinhead in crop braces and 'Tear here' tattoo is misleading, because violent attacks can come in all colours and forms. But psychopathic types, booze-fuelled but livid with rage, hot with fist and boot, can launch their assaults with bewildering alacrity. Often schooled in violence by the army or prison, they, as their tattoos often state, 'Don't care'. And the subjects of the physical attacks are often vagrants, who are brought into Casualty near to death. One of the lads who was finally convicted of the celebrated murder of Altab Ali in 1978 confessed, offhandedly, to some seventeen other attacks and talked lightly of killing or setting light to vagrants. There is sometimes a Nazi-ish pseudo-political rationale: the tramps are 'trash', human refuse who deserve elimination. But that's usually a rationale for their cowardice; the pissed vagrants are just easy pickings. Probably this level of violence is unremarkable compared with New York or Chicago, but violent assault for petty or non-existing motives is the meat and potatoes of the local police courts.

The tramp in the graveyard with the can of Brew is, however, a misleading stereotype, and general practice teaches you to expect drink problems in the most surprising places. The minicab supervisor with the beaming smile and the winning banter has a clank in her shoulder bag: it's the vodka she downs all day. A mother whose temper tantrums have the kids in fear and her husband sleeping out in the car is not depressed or menopausal after all, just half-cut all the time with gin she hides everywhere, even in the teapot. The solicitor's alcohol dependence is only picked up when, in hospital without booze for two days, she starts the DTs. And the skip driver who manages to fail an 8 a.m. breath test on the strength of his usual ten pints the previous night. And I am regularly surprised by patients I see drunk as lords at night who are devout abstainers in the surgery. Advising people is often complicated by the level of denial or, perhaps more generously, the mixed values people hold about drink, the 'I enjoy a drink, you get pissed, he's an alcoholic' outlook.

Heroin, on the other hand, is always seen as a dramatic shoot-up but is in fact more insidious, like soft snowflakes obscuring a windscreen. The old prewar stereotype was the medical addict: the respectable nurse or GP who had quietly become dependent through access to medical supplies. The next phase was the 1950s era of over-prescription by private GPs who were none too scrupulous about issuing prescriptions which were technically legal to people who said they were addicted. In theory, this was to prevent bona fide addicts from having to purchase their 'medicine' illegally and becoming further contaminated by the criminal world. Both implied a view of drug addiction as a disease which needed treatment by a doctor, rather than a decision or a series of personal and peer choices. And doctors prepared to prescribe were very widely, and perhaps knowingly, taken advantage of by people who often supplemented their legal supplies with illegal purchases or sold their surplus to live on.

Despite this, in a curious way, the 'British system', for a time, worked. Many 'registered' addicts, while making no serious attempt to reduce, remained stable, able to work and reasonably healthy on their NHS prescriptions. Heroin use, at least in East London, was confined to a small, rather elitist coterie known to the police, the GPs and each other. These old lags of the opiate world used to turn up regularly at the first practice I worked at in Bethnal Green, veins tattooed with hundreds of injection sites and often blue and blocked, faces gaunt and inexpressive. They were animated by one subject – their prescription. When that was under discussion, their faces were moved with a flicker of inner illumination, which went, as if a lightbulb had been switched off, on any other subject. While there would be ritual protestations about the desire to go straight, they were exactly that, ritual. Heroin was a career which defined friends, movements and interests. But it was no longer an euphoriant, and the sense of inviolability which makes the opiates such effective analgesics was no longer the source of much pleasure. It really was, in that classic 1950s slang, a habit; unobtrusive, insistent and, within the bohemian world, of not little status. The East London addicts I treated were either professional criminals or working-class intellectuals, people who read novels, appreciated and sometimes played jazz and dabbled in art.

Things changed as, in the 1970s, heroin became easier to obtain and cheaper. Now one often saw the relatives first, parents who were concerned about erratic behaviour or domestic thefts. People who came with drug problems to the GP, a small proportion of those in contact with the drug, were generally in their teens and inhaled rather than injected. There were now women as well as men, but usually white. While the older addicts had measured out their prescriptions in imperial grains, the addict of the 1980s calculated by the ten-pound bags. The scale of addiction was very much wider: heroin was easily bought in many East End pubs. Petty crime was the main source of income; it was possible to gauge the degree of addiction in terms of how many car radios had to be stolen per day to provide the required daily number of bags. The diamond-like shards of a smashed passenger window are a common sight in gutters. The cars are often broken into in broad daylight and the cassettes expertly dewired in seconds to become a kind of criminal hard currency. I've lost five in as many years and occasionally speculate if it's my own patients with 'a two-cassette habit' who have removed them. The younger heroin user is in some ways easier to help but in others more difficult. Their physical addiction is minor and they are less likely to have health problems than those who inject with syringes and are at high risk from HIV infection. But they are less likely to come back to appointments or stick with agreements because they have nothing to gain from seeing a doctor and can much more comfortably slip back into the easier world of their friendly neighbourhood dealer. Many heroin-dependent Londoners still work: lorry drivers, window cleaners, swimming pool attendants and security guards. They are often current or ex-heavy drinkers and are usually conversant with most other illicit drugs. Diagnostically 'poly-drug abusers', they are in fact bright, bored and, in the classic East End way, on the make. 'I could get anything you've got in there in an hour,' boasted one, waving at my medical supplies bag, a paragon of free market liberalism. 'I'd not bother if I had anything to do,' said another who had drifted into serious addiction, 'but I pass the dealer's house on the way home every night and H makes the video more interesting.'

But many who start on the Bacofoil do graduate to the needle, despite HIV. This is gravely denied, but many a scallywag 'Temporary Resident' from the Wirral or Edinburgh turns out to have a row of needle marks when you roll up their sleeves. These are the ones, chic in clothing, who have no fixed address or income and beg in Camden Market or solicit in Finsbury Park. And many of the younger East End addicts join up with them and clump together in squats or illegal occupations on rundown estates where there is a sympathetic local chemist and a cheap supermarket to stock up on pop and sliced bread. The chilling truth is that many of them will die before they decide to detox and that in the meantime the most important medical task is to keep them from sharing needles, unsafe sex, prison and crime. A hospital case summary I received in 1990 sums up the management problems.

REASON FOR REFERRAL:

This 25-year-old registered heroin addict and former prostitute was brought in by the police on a Section 136 having been found hanging off a third-floor balcony in a 'delirious state'.

History:

She said she had a number of recent social problems. She had recently been diagnosed as HIV+, she had just split with her boyfriend, her father had been told he had cancer, and she had severe suprapubic pain.

She was admitted on a Section 4. In Casualty she became quite violent and had to be held down and was given Haloperidol 20 mg im. We attempted to get her to the Psychiatric Intensive Therapy Unit but there were no free beds.

Unfortunately, during the hand-over she slipped out of the ward some hours after admission. The police were informed. On matters heroin-related, special pleading is . . . habitual. One needs to be persistently cynical about the motives of doctors, governments and law enforcement agencies in utilising drug scares: whether it be psychiatrists removing power from pharmacists in the late nineteenth century, dollar imperialists using it to justify their military presence, or *Sun* editorialists and Radio 1 DJs attempting to add a moral glaze to their otherwise banal and self-interested activities.

But 'moral panics' aside, there has, in the 1980s, clearly been a rise in the destructive use of opiates in the West – this even before the HIV virus gave its particularly lethal twist to the tale. And reasons are to be sought on a material rather than symbolic level: subsistence peasant farming in the Third World is now linked by jet travel and migration patterns to a new sort of urban underclass in the cities of the West. That sense of inviolability which makes diamorphine such a medical boon in terminal care is an unsurprising resort for this new urban poor, already disenfranchised from public life and low on personal dignity.

It's all too easy to mock Drugwatch, but what *is* to be done for the kids crashed out in the concrete stairways in a muddle of Bacofoil, Special Brew and misspelt graffiti? The Scottish New Town addicts trying to kick in an encounter group of elderly alcoholics, or the junkie parents whose child is drifting inexorably into neglect? The user-friendly agencies, the inner-city GPs organised and able to help, high-quality secondary inpatient care, including more appropriate psychiatric services, the sort of policing which would help communities threatened by drugs help themselves (as in Christiana and in Dublin), the training and educational opportunities to refill lives whose meaning has been gutted by drugs, even decent wages and staffing for the customs services – all these are being undercut by the general policies of a government which simultaneously expresses sanctimonious horror about heroin.

Heroin gets mixed up in crime (to pay for it) which thence becomes compounded by violence. So heroin users tend to present with wounds or evidence of assault (sometimes at the hands of the police, more often fellow addicts) as well as the medical complications of syringe use (local infections, septicaemias, renal, liver and cardiac valve disease, now Aids). Junkies are also seen by doctors as inherently 'manipulative' (not a useful word: almost everyone is manipulative about something, and being 'straightforward' is also a way of getting what you want). And, living in opiate time, they run habitually behind the clock and then belatedly expect instant service. But, all that aside, they are more rewarding to treat than some other categories of respectable patients.

The problems in the East End, in overall terms, are far greater with alcohol because it is *far* more widely and destructively abused, especially when it worsens personality disorders or mental illness. One is repeatedly faced with intoxicated patients who are also threatening, grandiose, or just impossibly demanding ('I need a full, typed medical report on my last beating for the Divorce Court this morning'). It is often taught that psychotics don't drink, tending to regress to an anti-life of wall-staring and roll-ups. But when they do, their drunkenness is wild and roaring, they are magnificently deluded. And, if lacking insight, hard to overawe, even to locate. The pattern here is for a patient who in the 1960s would have been cared for in an asylum which, if regimented, was at least warm, now to be discharged into 'community care'. This, in reality, means an otherwise unlettable council house, a giro and a two-weekly jab of depot-medication at the local Modecate Clinic. The active therapy which the critics of institutional neurosis in the old mental hospitals saw as the strength of 'community care' is largely lacking. A good day centre exists but there is only one, inconveniently located; and, without well-organised transport, it is impossible to guarantee attendance. So the stable, well-medicated and socially integrated dischargee easily loses momentum, not attending the day centre, missing the jab clinic, going wandering, his mental condition deteriorating often in antisocial ways.

Psychotic illness is a small part of the psychiatry of general practice; much more time is spent in dealing with less spectacular management of anxiety, depression, relationship problems and maturational crises. But the psychotics have such a powerful presence. Bromfield, the boy with voices who tell him bad things, rang me to inquire if the flicker in the table lamp could make him do evil. Winston James, with the magnificent brow and bearing, a Trinidadian Marx, imperious when mad, walking naked through tube trains, leaving his top-floor flat in blackened ruins while he strode the battlements and bayed at the moon. Mrs Montgomery, clad in black witch's clothing and clawing voice, who comes in every month for certificates even though they are valid for 'infinite time'. The meek chain-smoking St Lucian carpenter who set light to a hospital wing and whose son drowned himself at Margate. The garrulous Essex electrician who sometimes thinks he can speak eight languages and is in charge of tank divisions in Africa. 'Never mind the prickly heat,' he shouted when I last persuaded him in a minicab to go to the mental hospital. All five now in remission but their memory still potent: grandiose in flight, now grounded by their pills and long-acting depot injections they can't forget to take.

So it's the housing officer who might call you out to 'do something' about Mr C who is banging at night or whose bathroom taps have flooded the floors beneath or who has set light to his kitchen again. And you realise rather ashamed that you haven't seen Mr C even for his long-term sick notes. And that the last entry in

150

the notes was '? grandiose'. And Mr C is not in, or at least not answering. But through the kitchen window can be seen a charred kitchen, with electric oven still on, many packets of stale sliced bread and, yes, a litter of lager cans. And after a week of phone calls to the consultant and chases round the back of the estate, the British Transport police phone up from Swindon: 'We've got a naked chap on the platform, says he's God Almighty. Smells of drink but it's not just that.' So I next see Mr C in the back high-security ward of the mental hospital. His fine head is softer now as he shuffles into the interview room in slippers and dressing gown. On the ward two patients are arguing with themselves in quiet dementia; two others, a Sikh boy in a turban and hornrims and another lady with a crimson knitted cardigan which she incessantly twists, are being instructed by two nurses with a blackboard, something quite complicated that I can't understand. The other two nurses are in the office talking about their regrading applications and an unsatisfactory union meeting.

Mr C is morose. He wants to go back home. He says he will take the pills now. Insight! He has got better because he remembers he has to take the pills. But then he gets cross again. 'The consultant is mad. I'm the only one here who understands how things work.' I sign the Certifying Order for another month: he's better off here.

CHAPTER 10

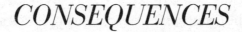

CONSEQUENCES

The medical familiarities: viral illnesses, repeat prescriptions, pregnancies gathering momentum, back-chat simultaneously banal and serious. But a normal East End day also includes dog bites, police assaults, drunken falls, carcinoma, methadone, TB and termination of pregnancy. A consultant writes, from the heart, 'Clinics are impossibly overbooked at the moment' and I spend twenty minutes trying to locate a registrar who will take responsibility for a patient who may need admission. All this is a condition of working in a health service in managed decline.

64 OM	82 Para 1
74 Scabies	83 TOP
79 TOP	88 CIN 3
80 TOP	90 NAI Case Con

A young Manchester boy is dragged in by his mum who thinks he's going crazy. While the boy sits unresponsive, almost gibbering, the mother explains that her son's spouse had twins and went into premature labour at thirty-two weeks. The children were delivered by caesarean section but both suffered anoxia and are severely brain damaged. The father managed to visit the Special Baby Unit a couple of times but one day couldn't take it any more and ran, from his wife, his children, from the north, from his future. One moment the father of two triumphant twins, the next, he stutters bitterly, 'a pair of spastics'. Outrageous fortune. He starts to sob; long, hard and deep.

'How was he?'
'Effing and blinding as usual. Don't want this, don't want that. I give him his present and he threw it on the floor. Two black nurses were kind to him. They picked up my present but it was broken. I went to cry in the toilet. When I went back he was asleep, as usual.'
This once fine man she was married to for forty years now dementing in a back ward for the senile.

A Somalian girl of seventeen studying English speaks thoughtfully and with sad emphasis first about a scar on her shoulder which had developed an ugly keloid and then the history of its acquisition. She had been stabbed by soldiers in the Civil War with a broken bottle when she tried, as a girl of nine, to prevent her mother's rape. In the further course of the war she had lost her entire family, her father a rebel soldier killed in action, her mother and two sisters killed in an aerial bombardment, brother executed. Tears begin to stream across her handsome brown high-cheeked face as she explains that they have no graves and she is not in contact with other relatives who might help her to locate them. Although she lives, unhappily, with a Somalian family in a council house in Bow, she avoids fellow Somalians. 'They remind me of the war,' she says and starts crying again. How many refugees are nursing their unknown pains in grim East End council houses? How much sadness has the East End had to house and heal over the years?

Immigrant is a senseless word: a vacuum label that serves to stop thought, a limbo bottle into which we can project all our uncertainties about the other, the

strange, the new, the different and the strange murder-
ousness which lies at the heart of our own 'civilisation'.
And immigrants are so dissimilar. Mr Uddin is from
Sylhet: small, demonstrative, gnarled in a handsome
sort of way and oblique in his methods. He has been
refused Panadol in the chemist and been given instead
the chemically identical product Paracetamol. He thinks
it's because of the Cuts, a phrase everyone in the East
End understands. 'The Cuts give me bad headache', an
inspired kind of metaphor perhaps. When he gets his
prescription, unctuous, saluting, grovelling, pressing
my hand to his forehead.

But young Miah is quite different: upstanding, direct,
rather take it or leave it. When I tell him it's his father's
nerves which are making him ill he understands, agrees
and wants to know why his father wasted so much
money on a second opinion in a private hospital. In his
eyes I can remember the rather distraught looks of his
father. 'Are you worried about anything?'
    'No, it's just the evening shift, I'm working at Dag-
enham now, mustn't be late.'
    Dagenham that vast factory-suburb to our east which
sucks in shift workers from all over London now assim-
ilates him into the stern disciplines of collective work,
unionism, overtime and industrial disputes. So different
to being the junior waiter in his uncle's Indian takeaway
in Chatham. He stands there, a dreamy boy born in a
land of lakes, in his Joe Bloggs track bottoms, asking
about his children's injections before haring off to Dagenham in his beat-up Cortina. He is the father now.
His kitbag has a Kiss FM sticker. 'Do you listen?' I ask.
'Yes, mate' with an ironic smile. 'It's the sound of
young London, innit.'

The LDDC, as usual, have done everything back to
front. First they let Olympia & York build their mono-
lith at Canary Wharf, then as the traffic jams and delays
become intolerable it occurs to them that services and

infrastructure, in particular road access, will be needed. So the Limehouse Link, an underground five-lane motorway of about three-quarters of a mile, has to be rammed through the main two Limehouse council estates in record time, demolishing a 500-foot tower block, obliterating 500 homes and requiring the compulsory rehousing of a further 2,000 people. All so that the journalists on the *Daily Telegraph* can get to work on time. The final stages of the 'decant' as it is called on St Vincent's Estate are nearly finished. Those who still hang on are drowned in dust, deafened by continual noise and pelted with debris from the never-ending convoys of haulage lorries. Visiting the last few patients waiting to be moved – a Bangladeshi boy with insulin-dependent diabetes, one of eleven people living in a two-bedroomed flat, a new birth visit for a mum of sixteen, a white-haired asthmatic squeaking and hissing even after the nebuliser – is like visiting the aftermath of a bombing raid. Blocks in which people have lived out sweaty, tempestuous and overcrowded lives are now so many heaps of rubble being picked and nipped at by disdainful cranes. A community which was so recently alive and kicking reduced to a range of brick mountains and foothills of bent wire and concrete. How easy it is for them to destroy. At least when the nineteenth-century equivalent of Olympia & York smashed their railways and 'sanitary improvements' through the East End rookeries they had a purpose, or at the lowest an excuse. But as far as I know there has been no recent outbreak of cholera in Limehouse and South Poplar.

When Jesse was six he entered a competition, well a PR stunt, for East End school children to draw their ideas for Canary Wharf, organised by Wayne Travelstead the previous developer. On canary yellow paper he drew a mixture of houses, offices and workshops with a drive-in cinema, ethnic food centres and a museum of the docks. Everyone got a free beach buggy to drive round the water's edge and cars were banned. Now thirteen, he goes with his friends on mountain bikes: 'It's weird, another city. A bit like New York. It won't be the East End any more.' He sounds quite pleased about this.

The 'Risby Three' were the last tenants to leave Risby House: one a patient of mine with myelopathy which was getting visibly worse with the strain, emotional and physical, which she was under as they first cut off the electricity, then the telephones then finally the water. From her eighth floor she had a marvellous view of the imperious motorway snaking through what had once been her neighbourhood and causing her home to be demolished. 'I can't hack it any more,' she wept. 'They keep on trying to give me money: "Why don't you go off to Portugal for a couple of weeks? The Algarve is very nice this time of year." As far as the LDDC are concerned we are just people getting in their way. And they are so pompous about it. But they still won't put the agreement they keep on about into writing. And I've no clothes, no phone, they've tinned up the doors and bust the lift.' Eventually, by sheer insistence, she got the transfer to a bungalow she wanted.

Others have been less ruthlessly dispersed: bribed to go off to Ireland, this a man with bone cancer who won't be able to get proper hospital treatment in Southern Ireland; another local community organiser bundled off to Essex with a part-paid mortgage; many families shunted down to Timber Wharves, a soulless fake-Georgian estate which the LDDC bought off the peg to house its displaced persons. One family even got their hands on a flat in the fine Georgian mansions which still line the Mile End Road. All in the process losing that sense of community which is one of our most precious possessions. 'So pompous, so much power': the refrain is haunting and ancient. Further St Vincent's laments; two legs broken in unfilled pot holes, builders always in a bad mood: just think we're in the way. Permanent grime even if you dust three times a day, pneumatic drilling which starts at 8.20, the roads closed, clogged and slippery with spilt excavation loads.

Obese slightly grim lady with a kidney defect which generates exquisitely painful stones admitted on Christmas Eve. 'The hospital, I can't say enough about it. The doctors dressed up as fairies, we had a service, pudding and carols. Thank God for the NHS, that's what I say.' What she doesn't know is that the day surgery wards have been padlocked till the end of the year and outpatients virtually closed for two weeks. Aim: to cut overspend; result: ever-lengthening waiting lists and pandemonium when the hospital reopens.

The end of term: a benign madness. Gayhurst School is a Victorian edifice whose gaunt outline lords it ecclesiastically over London Fields. It boasts outside toilets that freeze in the winter and a tough tarmac playground where boys bounce heaven and hell out of each other while girls angelically skip and pass comments. The children come from the local tower blocks and council houses; dads with tattoos and Silk Cut, young mums in leggings and Benidorm T-shirts, battered buggies, rusty Volvos, the playground a planned wargame of physical encounter. It provides a paediatric refresher course for any doctor chalking up the behavioural problems, the poorly nourished and the spotty, and monitoring the periodic outbreaks of resistant lice and road accidents inflicted by passing lorries and cars. This end of year is the worst ever for the staff: Tower Hamlets has newly taken over financial and managerial responsibility for the local schools from the ILEA. This immediately puts two terrific strains on the staff. They have to, somehow, reproduce locally the range of special resources formerly provided by the Inner London Education Authority and, worse still, do it on a budget which is raised locally. The poorest boroughs of inner London also have the highest fertility rates but since the 1920s have been subsidised by the ILEA levy which was raised London-wide and to which the very affluent boroughs contributed too. Now suddenly a borough which has difficulty cleaning its streets is meant to provide nursery, junior, secondary and adult education, including that for children with special needs, on a plummeting budget. No wonder at this time of year most headteachers' first job is to calm down the teachers who troop into their offices brandishing resignations.

My continuing correspondence with the Professor of Gastrointestinal Sciences: 'What worries me is that this process of de-civilisation of human relations in so many spheres is going on with the reluctant acquiescence of most of the "experts".' Actually the consultants don't have much stomach for the 'Reforms' either but are being blackmailed by the threat of complete withdrawal of capital funds if they don't 'opt out'.

The much-used and much-loved open air swimming pool whose tiled changing rooms and children's paddling pool have cooled generations of local children is now closed. 'Where's our f'ing swimming pool?' is scrawled discreetly over its entrance. Will 'Where's our f'ing education?' be written over the school gates before long? Parents collect for the Gayhurst carnival procession converging through the roars of the cowboy drivers of skip lorries, snappy dogs, roving drunks and broken glass. Some have cameras, all look weary and end-of-termishly subdued. Then suddenly the children emerge. Marvellous children transformed with masks and hats and plumes and costumes into Teenage Mutant Ninjahs, Robin Hoods, skeletons and Batwomen, luscious with hand-painted pearls, crowns of egg boxes and orbs of scrap metal.

The steel band hasn't arrived but the children dance a huge intricate costume barn dance with each other's finery: pirates with willow trees, ghosts with magic cats and princesses with rhinos. The many different nationalities protrude from the mask edges and cloak corners: these are African and West Indian and Asian Cockneys as well as whites. United in their infinitely complex play, curving and dancing in unsupervised grace with the costumes which they and their teachers and helpers have been constructing for weeks in wonderful, multicoloured, sequinned defiance of Tory sadism, Labour incompetence and parental gloom.

Canary Wharf is 'topped out' today. A helicopter persistently nibbles and buzzes at the pointed top of the 800-foot obelisk to photograph the lowering of a stainless steel pyramid cap by a roof-mounted crane. The cap, which glows a sickly gold colour visible twenty miles away, is garnished with large Canadian and British flags. Fat Canary is now the biggest building in Britain and the second biggest in Europe, forty-one feet below the Frankfurt Messeturm. It is the centrepiece of the £4 billion Olympia & York seventy-one-acre site, has utilised 27,500 tonnes of steel, 500,0000 bolts and is said to eventually employ 11,500 people.

'Fucking white elephant if you ask me,' says the manager of the local bank as he opens his shirt expansively in the Chinese restaurant. 'I mean if you're going to build a new town you do the roads and the sewers first don't you. And look at this place at night, there's more going on in Gravesend.' He knows about Gravesend, was assistant manager there, he tells his two juniors. He's fed up with the bank because he's quadrupled the business in ten years but they won't give him a profit share. Anyway there's a recession on and he doesn't like being responsible for calling in the receivers on his drinking mates. 'But my missus tells me, "You'll miss it like mad." I couldn't go back to being a nobody in a suit in Head Office.' He has another brandy while the under-managers tell him what a character he is. He laments that Sammy the Chinese owner isn't in tonight. The service would have been a bit sharper; 'He owes me, see.'

17 12 90 SHORT AUDIT OF TEMPORARY RESIDENTS

1	Housing problems	20	Glandular fever	38	Analgesia dependent
2	Bleeding piles	21	Contraception		
3	Asthma	22	Homeless (living in back of catering waggon)	39	Hypertensive lost pills
4	Stiff neck			40	Nervous debility
5	Otitis media			41	Schizophrenic; medication problems
6	? Appendicitis	23	Asthma		
7	Chickenpox	24	Worms		
8	URTI	25	Back pain	42	Neck pain
9	Flu jab	26	Pregnant	43	Acute chest pain
10	LRTI	27	Assault	44	Drug dependent ? HIV
11	LRTI (sedation refused)	28	Temazepam dependent		
12	Asthma	29	Warts	45	Certificate
13	Alcohol dependency	30	Hypertension; migrant worker	46	Alcohol problems
14	Alcohol dependency	31	LRTI	47	Asthma
15	DTs	32	Epistaxes	48	Lower abdo. pain, ? ectopic; homeless
16	Homeless	33	Otitis media		
17	Assault	34	Acute abdo. pain	49	Scabies
18	Alcohol problems	35	Dental abscess	50	OD
19	Hormone replacement therapy	36	Gastroenteritis		
		37	Asthma		54 per cent Homeless

I watch the topping-out from the top of a council tower block in Poplar, now a dwarfed giant. It had taken a long time to get past the entryphone where two labourers are struggling with pieces of steel lift carcass which are too heavy for them. 'Cunt, you shit yourself,' says one pair of straining legs from the lift as the steel they are grappling with slowly slips to the ground. The flat is dingy, cluttered and warm; through the net curtains there's a good view of the topping-out and the helicopter circling the tower. Mrs O'Rhiodan tried to come to surgery, her swollen feet went red and kept her awake for two nights. She lies under a blanket in the sitting room apologising. Why is the infection spreading? Too close to the gas fire, late onset diabetes, or the whisky nips she takes down in the 'Intrepid Prince'? She has a

160

prematurely lined face which is beautiful when animated and a rubicund sense of humour, eyes that have
twinkled too often for another round at closing time.

'What do you think about the tower?' I ask.

'Wouldn't like to do the window cleaning,' I think
she says. But she's talking about her windows which
have been up for double glazing for years. These flats
are like fridges in winter. I feel the window she's
waving at and my fingers sink into the rotting wood-
and-putty frame.

Her handsome husband, an unemployed ex-docker,
chats while I wait for the lift; 'She misses the old days,
we've no friends nowadays. No work either.'

'Well, I suppose they go together,' I offer.

This old ill woman is in her early fifties. The local
paper announces today that food is being given away
in Hackney; 'Each person will be entitled to a tin of
mince and a pound of butter.' But must bring pension
book or income support or family credit book. Five
hundred come to queue in the cold.

Mother of six, mid-thirties, one has cerebral palsy, now
she's got insulin-dependent diabetes and the latest one
looks a bit twitchy. She holds it with knowledgeable
affection. Her face since I have known her has become
softer and more beautiful. Today she is like a proletarian
Madonna as painted by Vermeer. I think the baby's all
right and she smiles silent relief.

The LDDC have a new prime-time TV advertisement
where computer-generated silhouettes of great cities –
Paris, New York, Sydney – are succeeded by an outline
of Docklands as a 'new world city'. Their marketing
manager spouts clichés: 'Billions invested . . . over
200,000 will soon work here . . . good-quality life-style
facilities . . . waterfront locations.' And a new poster
has gone up for people to read as they fume in the
Commercial Road's permanent traffic jam: 'Shouldn't
London be a better place to work in? Well in 48 weeks

it will be.' But as I drive back through Marsh Wall, the toytown Docklands Light Railway is out of service and down at South Quay Plaza the only action is a queue of hard-hats and clerks at a sandwich shop. If this is a new world city then the newspaper kiosk at Chancery Lane tube station is Cincinnati.

The next stop is a new birth visit, for an anxious young mother who had worried throughout her first pregnancy. She is asleep and her mum conveys me past a posse of growling alsatians and a group of chain-smoking relatives watching *Neighbours*. The TV is covered with vast, pink, quilted congratulation cards of the sort East Enders prefer for first babies. 'She's very down,' her mum, a depressive, assures me. But she's not: sooty-headed, milk-faced and lazy-limbed in a double bed beside her daughter, she smiles and stretches with satisfaction. I half examine, half cuddle the child, flesh 'so dear achieved', proud too.

Chinese schoolgirl with asthma. It's got worse in the freezing fog. She splutters and coughs as she sets out to school in the morning. 'Don't like them silly puffers,' she says in purest Cockney.

'Well tough because you've got to use them.'

Her mum still can't get the hang of English but she's bright, inquiring and, in the East End idiom, articulate.

'What do you like at school then?'

'Algebra's best, but we ain't had a maths teacher for two months.'

Baby clinic: the children of Docklands come for their tests and their jabs: alert, innocent, growing bodies. A nine-week-old, late for his check, endearingly pisses over my shirt and the couch. His mum comforts her other mischievous son, a proletarian 'Just William', as he tries not to cry when he has his jab.

In the evening surgery the London poor who dwell in the shadow of Docklands' new pinnacle of success troop in.

CONSEQUENCES

A pair of asthmatic girls, the younger with only half the lung capacity she should have and with her growth already stunted, their inhalers under-used as usual. They must both start a course of steroids. 'Wot Ben Johnson took?' says little Jade, interested.

Deep in the computer, I think for a moment I've heard Ben Jonson's name; Jonson the Stepney dramatist, bon viveur and bricklayer, who wrote that great satire on monetarism, *Volpone*, set in Venice, the most acquisitive, glittering and corrupt city of its day, the Manhattan of the Renaissance. How he would have loved the argots of the modern poor and laughed at the LDDC. As he wrote:

> What a rare punishment
> Is avarice to itself?

Billy Watson hobbles in: 'I was ten times better when I was on the drink and the fags.'

An Irish would-be taxi driver comes in for the medical which they must do before embarking on the Knowledge. It should cost £25 and he has applied to the Dole for it but, since he's been unemployed three years, they have nothing to offer but 'a scheme'. His mother was in the previous night to plead for him. We do it for half-price. He has perfect sight.

A missionary from a Nonconformist tabernacle comes in complaining of exhaustion: he has been doubly bereaved, flat broken into and last had a holiday two years ago. His eyes radiate a baffled decency, his clothes cheap and hard-worn.

An Asian boy has broken his shoulder playing football. He goes to a hard, mainly white school in Poplar where football is how boys prove themselves. What passion must have gone into that challenge? He needs a note because the police picked him up when he was coming home early because of the pain. His mate got

163

taken to the station. He talks of the police as remote, cruel, unreasonable . . . already.

Then a married lady who needs the Morning-After Pill after a fling. 'Perhaps you're in love?'

'Well, I got a bit carried away, didn't I? But it's nice after all the years of not being wanted when someone cares for you.'

An Irish building worker in the Blackwall Tunnel maintenance works, shows me a dental abscess which is oozing creamy yellow pus and tells me Blackwall Tunnel jokes. He and his family have come recently from Belfast and, always with a charming smile, he declines to tell me why. One of the off-duty receptionists phones up, worried about Mrs O'Rhiodan; 'I'm going to go over myself and give her a bread poultice.'

Proletarian decency over monetarist efficiency: one driven by compassion and the solidarities of work and neighbourhood, the other by the simpler calculation of profit and loss. There is no physical monument to what generations of decent working-class East Enders have created and given and made and suffered. But César Pelli the architect of the Fat Canary tells us that 'A skyscraper recognises that by virtue of its height it has acquired civic responsibilities. We expect it to have formal characteristics appropriate for this unique and socially charged role.' Now they would be interesting to see.

Micky the bookie breezes in to stock up on pills. Always a bit dashing he shocks me with his health. Nearly a year ago I'd finally persuaded him to let me examine his rectum and had hit a craggy mass three centimetres up from the anus. We were talking about the Ascot Gold Cup only the conversation lagged a little as I tried to manoeuvre him round to try and palpate bi-manually. 'Have you ever thought of wrestling?' he suggested unkindly. At first thought inoperable, he'd had an eight-hour procedure while two teams of surgeons resected the tumour. He's nearly died twice, lost six stone and been too weak to leave home for two months. And here he is again, gaunt but newly handsome like a 1950s Hollywood film star, his eyes moist and vivid. 'Now give me plenty of those bowel tablets, I can't be rushing off to the loo every ten minutes. There's too many thieves about, both sides of the counter.' He takes two four times a day and I write a scrip for 300.

'I'll see you again in about a month then, Mr Burroughs.'

'Ok, Dave, see you in thirty-seven and a half days.'

A gay shop assistant at Harrods. Worried in a mock-offhand way about a persistent sore throat. Much unsaid. He's reading Andrew Holleran's novel about the Fire Island days and we talk about that instead. Five years ago there were half a dozen HIV patients at the London Hospital, now there are over a hundred with fourteen new patients every quarter. Three East London doctors have died of Aids. Today two heterosexuals requested HIV testing. 'This could be the most important day in my life,' said one as I took the specimen. And still the USA spends more in a minute on military defence than it does in a year on Aids research and treatment. An anonymous doctor writing in the *BMJ* about medicine in Central Africa reports that over half the occupants of his hospital's beds are HIV positive.

Go to not pay my poll tax in the new marble-fronted magistrates court in Bow Road. Don't know what to expect but there are 400 of Hackney's refuseniks packing out the waiting rooms; white working-class families who have come in minicabs waving fags and summonses, rampacked E8 Jamaican families, grizzled dads in black leather pork-pie hats, elder children in trainers and leather blousons. When the tannoy asks if anyone has changed their mind and now wants to pay up, there is a great roar of mirth, defiance and cries of 'Rasclat'.

SOME LIVES!

I walk home through Bow, stronghold of Tower Hamlets 'Liberals': face-lifts and flower baskets everywhere
but half the shops in the Roman Road have their leases
up for sale. A row of new terrace houses is half built
and left derelict; presumably the Housing Association's
funds ran out. Victoria Park has suffered an outbreak
of royalism with illuminated coronets over its pompous
new main gates. To pay for this royal blue clap-trap
they have had to close the swimming pool.

Bank messenger reminisces about the old Lloyds building. 'All bronze scallops everywhere. They cleaned the
chandelier twice a year and it took four men to lower
it on the pulley. Got bought by a hotel in Italy. Don't
see anyone wanting to buy the Richard Rogers rubbish.'
I would. Its savage blue night-light is the most beautiful
thing in the London night.

After a clear-out at home bring in a box full of
children's books for the waiting room. They'll be taken,
of course, but that's predictable and at least they will
provide some enjoyment in the meantime. The next
night I find a Noddy book being avidly read by a
woman of twenty-three.

Bach's *Christmas Oratorio* in the cold stone of Christ
Church, Spitalfields. Eighteenth-century music in
eighteenth-century London. The church is crammed,
the unamplified singing in German deeply moving,
yearning with the full depth of Bach's religious conviction. The sound hangs in the clerestory, moves round
the entablature and is stilled against the buttresses. One
is transformed for a moment to a devout burger of
Protestant Leipzig. Outside the beggars are eighteenth-
century too, twisting creatures in rags, clawing the
best opportunity of bourgeois custom for a while with
curses and imprecations before they return to their skips
in the sleet.
    Later in the week I visit a newborn child with croup

166

and her sixteen-year-old mother in an unlit room full of Christmas squalor. The baby is fat and breathes with difficulty, the carpet is sticky and the phone cut off. The Evangelist's words, 'Das kinder is lieben', hang grimly over this proletarian nativity.

The road pushes on. It's like a gold rush whose prospectors wear hard-hats but are burrowing away at various heights with the focused passion of gold-diggers. The sun gleams off their bright moulded helmets as they seem to nudge and chatter with their pneumatics, climb and fall on crane hooks and hurtle dump trucks honking and farting round the stanchions of the light railway. Everywhere is activity: high in the distance on the sky-blue-clad edifice of Canary Wharf the steel erectors can just be seen bolting girders into ascending shape, a procession of heavy lorries queue in coils by the new roundabout, as big as Hyde Park Corner, taking their turn to empty rubble, in the foreground the demolition workers prise and lever apart the roof of 'Charlie Brown's' public house.

'Charlie Brown's', one of the most famous of the Dockland pubs whose landlord built up his own menagerie by swapping sailors' pets for drink on tick. I remember 'Charlie Brown's' awash with morning dockers off shift in marching squadrons, shouting and smiling and gulping down foaming beer. I have a cherished old photo of Francis Bacon drinking in the pub with sailors in uniform. The pub was full of the promise of the day, as early morning pubs in sunlight are: full of prospects, possibilities. But since the docks closed, the pub has been in limbo, dog-eared, uncared for, usually empty except for an odd crowd of CID men celebrating a birthday or a conviction, or a curious tourist. Now it's crashing down while behind it grows a new East End Manhattan served by great curled intersections of concrete and beneath it a new six-lane underpass is set to rumble.

At lunch hour, the old Chinese street of Pennyfields is crowded with building workers drinking milk and eating hot dogs from a street corner stall, sprawling in the sun with long hair and short trousers. They are like industrial Vikings and at their waists dangle girdles which contain their scaffolding tools and designate their trade. They lie akimbo: tired and proud, looking up at what they have built in a kind of daze. A Chinese cook comes out from behind the restaurant to pour away slops and contemplates them gravely. From the gutter a tramp, coats tied with string, mimes reading from a yellowed newspaper held in mittened hands. I watch the incessant cranes from the window of a maisonette in Pennyfields full of faded photographs of various popes, a lumpy brown sofa and heaps of closely annotated racing papers. Says O'Hagan, 'To look at these pills anyone would think that I'm sick.'

O'Hagan, a lifelong hypochondriac, now has cancer spreading, despite various chemotherapeutic batteries, from his prostate to his hips and spine. A small pungent skin secondary has burgeoned on the nape of the neck which we are discussing evasively. He has a table strewn with pills which we are marking up: 'For Pain', 'For Sleep', 'For Nerves'. He is not without a certain satisfaction and has deep brown eyes, a face which is increasingly gaunt and sallow and a small unpleasant dog who I insist is excluded from our consultation.

'It's half of Ireland out there, you know. I see 'em in the "Rose and Crown". "A pint of Guinness please." "No make that three." We built the docks and now we're knocking them down.'

He's been bribed to move out of the way of the road, given a deposit for a bungalow in Tralee; 'But I don't trust the health service out there, or what is left of it.'

Instead the family have sent a nephew, a quiet man, to be with him as he dies.

O'Hagan and I were enemies or at least had opposing views on the severity of his complaints for years but the arrival of this illness has made us intimates, him slightly teasing of my newfound concern, me guilty. We sit complaining about the dust and the noise and the road and the men with helmets and naked kneecaps. I think he secretly relishes the activity, the relentlessness and the circulars about double glazing. Not so the older Cockney ladies who now talk of Limehouse-before-the-Road in pre-lapsarian terms. 'And they told us such lies . . . I'm eating dust!'

There was a meeting in the local hall to which the junior surveyors were sent to answer questions. An ex-dustman reported proudly that the language had been exceptionally colourful, 'Especially the birds'.' There had been a chant, just like football, 'We don't want to see the shit, we want to see the governor.' Because as a more proper lady had told me, 'Mr Reichmann isn't over here getting all the dust.' An old docker told me that he never went down there any more, 'It makes me sick in the heart. That yuppie-town, I can't take it. Do you know they've even tried to take my sister's parking space away. Born, bred and ten years saving for her own car and now she's got to be charged all of a sudden.'

Said a cleaning lady, 'That tunnel, it's not for the likes of us. And it should have gone under the river anyway. Why disrupt our lives for years so stock-brokers can drive to work.'

Mr Wade and his wife spent New Year's Eve listing all the firms that used to operate on the Island. 'They done it all too fast. I don't see it working myself.'

It's not, unfortunately, that people have a political hostility to capitalism or the City; East Enders have serviced and do service the Golden Mile in every capacity from broker to tea lady. They just want it to leave them alone.

'That's the trouble with us,' said a bright-eyed ex-munitions worker. 'We Cockneys think we're so tough but we get taken for a ride because we want to believe.

SOME LIVES!

I mean during the Blitz, there we were squatting in silly little trenches in Victoria Park and when it rained we put our umbrellas up. Because they told us it was all right. But it wasn't. But they wouldn't have won that stupid war without us.'

CHAPTER 11

———◦⊙◦———

ACROSS FIVE OCEANS

The writer Darcus Howe describes the imaginary first day in London of an Icelandic tourist who is served coffee by a Punjabi in the Heathrow Airport canteen, passes schools in Slough where half the kids are Asian and West Indian, is conducted by a Nigerian on to a tube train, sprains his ankle which is examined by a Gujerati doctor and is taken home by a Cypriot minicab driver to watch Trevor McDonald report fighting between young West Indians and police in Liverpool. Darcus, a Trinidadian Londoner, is himself an amalgam. I remember seeing him in August 1977 up a lamp post in New Cross, manoeuvring crowds of demonstrators to block the National Front's unwelcome passage as if he was setting a Lords outfield, and prowling over the stage at the old Naz cinema in Brick Lane denouncing the bishops and instructing the Bangladeshi kids, who couldn't follow his patois, 'to mek stand' for themselves. 'He's so anti-racist, he's gone to the other extreme,' muttered a local Labour councillor.

'It's all very well but they are taking over everything. And why do they get all the fuss? We can't get our community centre either. It's because we're white, that's our trouble,' the old hacks of East London Labour used to groan in those days – themselves, like as not, descendants of immigrants.

171

'Everything's changed. It isn't like it used to be,' is the universal *pietas*.

And, of course, it is. Immigrants have always come to the East End, partly because the port landed them there, but also because the area was outside the commercial jurisdiction of the City and the ecclesiastical control of the Bishop of London. Page one of the burial register of the Limehouse Church of St Anne's, next to my surgery, records in 1730 that the first men buried were an Asian seaman, John Mummud, two negroes called Christopher Hutton and Devonshire, then Jerimiah Orbeck, a Dane, and two Venetians. As a later rector wrote, 'Limehouse Churchyard is a sleeping world in miniature.' And the East End is five continents, a hundred mother-tongues and every skin colour a dermatologist could dream of. And the new arrivals have always been unpopular at first.

The sixteenth-century migrant Flemish brewers, who used hops instead of malt and ministered to London's thirst when wine was made pricey by the French wars, were immediately accused of the most terrible of London crimes, watering the beer. When the French silk-weavers came in the seventeenth century, establishing Spitalfields as a centre of fabric manufacture, the topographer Maitland complained, 'It is an easy matter for a stranger to imagine himself in France,' and anti-French rioting occurred whose slogans were jingoistic but whose cause was economic resentment by journeymen weavers.

In 1687 a Stepney rector wrote of the Huguenots, 'This set of rabble are the very offal of the earth who cannot be content to be safe here from the injustice and beggary from which they fled, and to be fattened on what belongs to the poor of our own land and to grow rich at our expense, but they must needs rob us of our religion too.'

By the mid-eighteenth century, there were also clearly defined East End Irish communities: the coal-heavers of Ratcliff, the labourers who cut the Rotherhithe Tunnel and built the first docks in Poplar, agricultural workers in the farms of Hackney. Driven from their native land by famine and grateful for even the lowest London wages in comparison with what they had suffered at home, they were blamed for every crime, major or minor. In their cottages in the Cable Street area, nicknamed 'knockvargis', they were assumed to be 'mumpers' (scroungers). Excluded from more skilled labour by trade restrictions, they did the dirty work and were then called dirty. Rather than organising with them against the employers, in particular the church builders who deliberately took on Irish labourers at half wages, established East End builders rioted against the Irish pubs in 1736 and had to be dispersed by the militia. The later Gordon Riots, in 1780, again nominally anti-Catholic, were often economic.

The East European Jews escaping the tsarist pogroms of the late nineteenth century were stigmatised as pedlars, as undercutters, as both work-shy and over-industrious, and blamed for disease and 'making alien' a Whitechapel which was, as usual, in permanent flux. A Stepney basket-maker is quoted by Mayhew in 1871: 'The more there goes away, the more there comes to fill the gaps. See here now, sir. Last month about five hundred was shipped off to Horsetrailier. Well, thinks I, good riddance. But last week there come about a thousand from abroad, an' they all landed at the docks, an' here they seem to stick, and it's mostly Polish Jews, they are.'

But perhaps most unfairly persecuted were the mid-twentieth-century migrants from Bangladesh who found their way to the East End through the shipping lines and went to work in the clothing trade and the restaurant business. Ironically they have, through the British East India Company which colonised Bengal and in the process destroyed its high-quality fabric industry, a long historical connection with the East End, unlike the Huguenots who had to leave France at

173

short notice to whatever destination they could find. And unlike, say, the Southern Irish, the Bengalis had a long record of fighting and dying for the British Empire, many drowning unnamed in German torpedoing of the merchant fleet which was the supply lifeline in the Second World War.

Probably, like so many migrants, the Bangladeshis did not plan to immigrate at all but to raise money in England to increase their family landholdings at home. But, forced into rotting overcrowded housing, they were duly accused of multi-occupation; working twelve-hour shifts they were said to be scroungers; devoted to family life (Spitalfields has the lowest proportion of single-parent families in Tower Hamlets) they were accused, as was every immigrant group, of taking the heart out of the East End. In fact they probably put it back. But being black, it has been impossible for them to slip into the mainstream of London society unnoticed (as to a remarkable degree the Huguenots and, much more slowly, the Irish and Jewish have done). They have had to take the blame and pain head on and have probably faced in total more assault and battery than sustained in the anti-Papist and anti-Semitic rioting. The most recent arrivals have been refugees from the civil war which broke out in Somalia in 1988, taking shelter with the small but significant Somali community which has been in Tower Hamlets for more than a hundred years. Many are women who have lost their husbands in the war and who have themselves been tortured, raped, or made to witness executions by the Barre regime. Often they are technically stateless or awaiting categorisation, which means they are without passport and papers and so cannot obtain benefits or housing to which they are entitled.

But it is migration that has always made the East End the most cosmopolitan quarter of London. The eighteenth-century East Enders would have been accustomed to Spaniards in red shirts, blue trousers, knife and earrings, big flaxen Swedes, Yankees with their felt hats, and lascars in fez and dungarees. Pierce Egan, in his 1873 *Life in London*, describes a Victorian East End knees-up as follows:

> Lascars, blacks, jack tars, coal-heavers, dustmen, women of colour, old and young, and a sprinkling of the remnants of once fine girls, etc., were all jigging together.

While Thomas Burke, in the 1928 *Limehouse Nights*, describes Mohammed Ali on the steps of the Asiatics' Home, 'swearing richly, with a feeling for colour and sting, strong in the vivid adjective . . . in a bastard dialect compounded of Urdu, Chinese and Cocknese'. The East End has both shaped generation after generation of migrants and been itself remade by their transitions. Immigrants, seamen, émigrés and exiles have stamped the area with a multiracial and nonconformist character which could neither be blitzed nor redeveloped out of existence. Its streets, its argot, its physiognomy and its habits are marked by journeys made across the globe to it and through it.

The Huguenots were not only the first but one of the most successful of immigrants into East London. 'Huguenot' is in fact a pejorative term, a corruption of the old Swiss-German word *eidgenosse*, meaning clique, just as 'Quakers' were so called because of their alleged twitching fanaticism, and 'Methodists' for their imagined strictness. French Protestantism, although legally tolerated since 1598, had been subject to intermittent persecution. The 'Chambre Ardente' of Henry II sentenced more than 500 Protestant heretics to death and the Massacre of St Bartholomew in 1572 was effectively a pogrom after the open-air marriage of Henry of Navarre, when Catholic Parisians killed 3,000 Huguenots. Subsequent massacres in Bordeaux and Lyons claimed a further 10,000 lives. Huguenots were excluded from various trades, their children were encouraged to leave home and enter Catholic convents, and, after 1600, they were subjected to 'dragonnade' when their households would be forced to billet soldiers, who were both costly to provide for and encouraged to abuse their hosts. While the majority stuck it out in France and worshipped in secret meetings known as *'désertes'*, echoing the Israelites suffering in the wilderness, migration to London had begun before the Edict of Nantes, which had guaranteed religious toleration, was repealed in 1685.

The repeal put tremendous pressure on French Protestants to repudiate their faith and make expedient conversions. The penalties were severe: although priests were allowed two weeks to leave the country, any lay Protestant found trying to escape was sentenced either to the galleys (if male) or to the convent for life. The majority abandoned their religion and made formal conversions. Exit routes needed to be both secure and able to transmit assets. Those leaving must have been people of tremendous commitment and courage. About a quarter of the émigrés came to England, with other big groups going to Switzerland and Germany, and smaller migrations to Ireland, the Cape of Good Hope and North America. The English émigrés were generally skilled craftsmen and, in London, were divided between weavers centred in the East End at Spitalfields and the manufacturers of more sophisticated luxury goods who, in Soho, were exempt from some trade restrictions and had ready access to the fashionable market of the Court. They were offered official refuge by Charles II, and public collections which raised large sums of money preceded their arrival. They were offered full naturalisation in 1709, despite protest from those London manufacturers whose own trade was threatened.

Although suppliers of the eighteenth-century equivalent of status symbols to French-imitating English fops, the Huguenots' ethos was of an austere democratic church with no elevation of priest and with simplified ceremony. In the 'Hog Lane' picture, Hogarth contrasts the plain Huguenot worshippers with both the overdressed French-imitating trendies and the loutish English commoners. Above them flies the kite which symbolises the Huguenot flight. The black character in this picture, as well as an erotic counterpoint to the etiolated fops, is also painted as a man of dignity, dressed as well as, if not better than, the white revellers in the pub. Ironically, the church from which the worshippers emerge was in reality once the property of a Greek-Christian congregation (known as *L'Eglise des Grecs*). Many of the Spitalfields Huguenots had moved from manufacture into property by the end of the eighteenth century. The fine plates used in church for the collection are still well preserved. Alms-giving was important, and many charitable organisations were financed by the émigrés, including 'La Soupe' in Fleur-De-Lis Street in Spitalfields, a 'maison de Charité'. A printed 'portion ticket' entitled the bearer to 'a pan of good broth mixed with six ounces of bread and half a pound of meat and the same weight of good bread', more nutritious than the modern equivalent.

It is therefore conventional to see the French Protestants as an industrious bourgeoisie who rapidly entered the English professional middle classes *en bloc*. Their religious fortitude as well as their manufacturing skills were well regarded. Although people like Defoe complained, they soon achieved affluence and thence assimilation. It was uncommon for them to speak French after 1775, although in Soho they were joined by later Roman Catholic émigrés and the French language persisted. Some of the best-known Huguenot innovation was, literally, new technology: the first operative obstetric forceps, glasses by the pioneer Dolland (who formed the contemporary High Street chain Dolland & Aitchison), the mapper and rococo engraver Rocque (now absurdly celebrated in a pricey nouvelle cuisine brasserie in one of the office developments which are obliterating old Spitalfields), and gun- and glass-makers more sophisticated in technique than their English rivals. An English observer wrote admiringly: 'They

177

confine themselves to their own business which they pursue with admirable address and skill to the great advantage, not only of themselves, but of the nation in general.' Although specifically excluded from banking in France, once in London many moved smoothly into the City, insurance, financial journalism, even the printing of bank notes, with an efficiency which has parallels with the nineteenth-century Anglo-Jewish establishment. Indeed, the Huguenots sound as conservative as the 'old establishment' that now gathers at the Garrick Club, named after the Huguenot actor-manager who was such an effective partisan of Shakespeare.

Yet we know far less of the humbler weavers from northern France who, excluded from the '*Grande Fabrique*' in Lyons, nevertheless made the wealth of the large Huguenot masters who built the grand houses off Brick Lane, now refurbished so exquisitely. The journeymen had often arrived in London via Amsterdam and Canterbury, had larger families, worshipped in East London less fashionably but no less devoutly and spoke French for longer. It was they who discovered how to give taffeta lustre and how to design and pattern brocade and who extended the street system east to Whitechapel and north to Bethnal Green. Were they among the 'Spitalfields mobs' who raged against the East India Company's illegal import of calico in the 'Calico Riots', who protested against the smuggling of cheap French silk, who swept down Piccadilly in conflict with their masters over a cut in wages, and who gave out cockades and broadsheets inscribed 'Wilkes and Liberty' and smashed the engine looms brought to Bishopsgate in 1769? One of the weaver-agitators in the loom riots has a French name, the other Irish: John Valline and John Doyle. They both were hanged outside the 'Salmon and Ball' in Bethnal Green Road despite protests and attempts at rescue. 'The unhappy sufferers,' wrote one observer, 'were therefore obliged to be turned off before the usual time allowed on such occasions, which was about eleven o'clock, when after hanging about 50 minutes they were cut down and delivered to their friends.'

Clearly the eighteenth-century East End mob was used on occasions as a stage army by employers and property owners, of whom Wilkes was the most brilliant tactician. But these explosions were also fuelled by a desire to get even with the rich and made East London's reputation for riot and lack of deference. 'The Spitalfields silk weavers and their apprentices had been long known for their anti-authoritarian turbulence,' writes E. P. Thompson in *The Making of the English Working Class*. The popular radicalism of men like Valline and Doyle who broke silk looms *en masse* was akin to those who hurled down enclosure fences or set fire to ricks. For these Spitalfields weavers, unlike the elite of Huguenot bankers, the soldiers and accoucheurs, were artisans; articulate but collective in their outlook. And for this reason Pitt's agents were sent to spy, especially in Spitalfields.

It thus can be said that the first wave of mass immigration into the East End accelerated social and political change on several levels. It set up what was effectively London's pioneer industrial suburb, and its artisan radicalism led to the foundation of modern working-class education and political organisation: 'a halfway house in the emergence of popular political consciousness', as Thompson puts it.

In eighteenth-century London emigration was as important as immigration, either through forced transportation to the penal colonies of America and Australia, or as an attempt to escape desperate poverty in Britain. The rise of industrial capitalism was achieved only by the degradation of the urban poor and the ruin of the London casual labourer. As the new rich moved elegantly west in those squares, parks and streets which Nash bolted together as soundly as a jobbing plumber, the East End rotted in its lawless jerry-built rookeries. Before the great nineteenth-century sanitary clearances, Covent Garden, Holborn and Blackfriars were workers' quarters as well as the East End where overcrowded artisans rented a share of a room close to their workplace. Child labour, orphan-snatching and drunkenness were facts of life. Blake's 'chartered streets' belonged to the merchants and industrialists now, nowhere more than in East London. Life was made bearable by gin, London-manufactured and therefore carrying no import duty and a profitable use of grain surpluses. A new ruling class who wanted to display their new wealth were cheek by jowl with the desperately poor, (although there was 'privatised' security in the form of narks and thief-takers).

With neither poor relief nor police, a crime wave was inevitable. To stem it, capital offences were enlarged, hanging made a public act of retribution and transportation introduced. Forgers, beggars, thieves, poachers, or rick-burners could be sentenced to death. If not hanged, they were sent to jails which were privately owned, charged for everything, and were, as now, overcrowded. Transportation was thought to demonstrate mercy (the prisoner was kept alive) but got rid of the need for prison and sent the prisoner to build an empire in conditions no free colonist would tolerate. So, until a combination of Independence and black slavery cut off the outlet, the American colonies were used. Then convicts were stowed in 'the Hulks', old troop transports moored and used as prisons off the naval ports and in the Thames Estuary. And finally, the ultimate weapon, Botany Bay. There is no doubt that many modern Australians and North Americans are children of the eighteenth-century East London tenements.

Victorian East London's chief immigrants were Jewish, and the Jewish presence is still strong and vivid. Not just the conventional loci: the Brick Lane bagel shop where Jewish taxi drivers from Ilford gather in the small hours for refreshment, Blooms Restaurant with its decrepit car park full of luxury saloon cars owned by successful ex-East Enders going down

Memory Lane, the smoked salmon curers in Assembly Passage or Gardiners Corner, now a strange white cylindrical building called the Sedgewick Centre but where, in 1936, Mosley's fascist march was stopped by mass street fighting. Rather it is something in the air: a particular cynical urban humour, a respect for education and for trade unionism, a sense of decency which survived the crucible of the slums of the late nineteenth century to overcome anti-Semitism and recover dignity and self-respect after the horrors and debasement of the East European pogroms. And it is the East End Jewish proletarians who didn't leave for Finchley and Woodford, the Minnies and the Stans and the Harrys and the Zeldas, who still make a rich and fascinating leaven in the East End of today.

It is a legacy which is highly political. Not only did Jewish refugees in London face the general resentment of the xenophobes, but to it was added the particular yoke of anti-Semitism. And the conflict of class interest which was present between the Spitalfields master weavers and their out-workers was felt much more sharply between the Anglo-Jewish establishment, already well integrated into the English bourgeoisie, and the poverty-stricken East European proletarians who flocked to the East End in flight from the great ukases of the tsar in the late nineteenth century. The twin pressures were to produce a powerful reaction, a Jewish radicalism specific to the East End and revolutionary in character, which was to make an impact on British communism and socialism.

The East End Jews were also responsible for a particularly rich vein of urban literature which, from Zangwill and Leftwich to Kops, Mankowitz and Wesker, is some of the best writing about the horrors and joys of living in the modern city in English literature. And, perhaps more importantly in establishing a modern British identity, the spread of mass-produced fashion garments through popular retail chains and the pioneers of popular culture in jazz, the music hall, even

Hollywood. The East End was the birthplace of Ronnie Scott and the Grade brothers, first debut of Chaplin, as well as the spiritual home of Tesco.

The medieval Jewish settlement was in the area of Old Jewry in the heart of the City, just west of where the Bank of England now stands. Without many legal rights, its inhabitants, who never exceeded 5,000, were subject to arbitrary imprisonment and mob violence from which they periodically sought sanctuary in the Tower of London. In a pogrom on the day of Richard I's coronation in 1189, thirty Jews were burnt alive in their houses or beaten to death on the streets. In 1210 all wealthy Jews in England were imprisoned pending investigation into their financial affairs; many were hanged and universal fines caused many to leave the country. And after further legal and physical attacks, Edward I expelled the Jews from England in 1290, by legend at least one ship on which they left being put aground and robbed in the Thames Estuary. The first Jewish cemetery in the Barbican, granted in 1177, was desecrated and its headstones used to repair Lud Gate.

The small Jewish community which remained were Sephardis who should have been entitled to call themselves Portuguese or Spanish; under the eye of the Inquisition, they had converted and been forcibly integrated. It was these survivors who successfully petitioned Cromwell during the Commonwealth for permission to celebrate Jewish rites openly again and reopen their own burial grounds. The first synagogues and burial grounds of the Resettlement were located on the border of the City and the East End (at Creechurch Street and Brady Street). Immigration restarted in the eighteenth century from Europe, in part because there was no specific legislation curtailing Jewish life in London. The Sephardic Jews were associated with integration and financial success; the newer Ashkenazi immigrants from the ghettoes of Germany, Poland and the Netherlands were less prosperous, establishing themselves first in the diamond, jewellery and watch trade in the Aldgate area. Ashkenazi migration increased after persecution in Bavaria, Bohemia and Moldavia during 1744, and the Great Synagogue was established in Aldgate in 1690. (It was destroyed in the Blitz in 1941.)

By 1791 there were said to be 11,000 Jews in London, polarised in class and geography between the respectable, conservative and assimilated West End Anglo-Jewish establishment like the Montefiores and the Rothschilds, and a largely poorer class of more recent Austrian and north German immigrants in the East End, artisans, tailors, street traders and small businessmen. Petticoat Lane, which owed its name to the French silk-weavers' staple product, was in fact, by the late eighteenth century, largely a market for secondhand clothes whose domination by Jewish traders was reflected in its Sunday opening. The faith here was often ultra-Orthodox and the labour hard; 'No work on the Sabbath and no rest on weekdays'. Zangwill, in *Children of the Ghetto*, describes the ultra-Orthodox Jews of the East End as 'Strange exotics in a land of prose, carrying with them through the paven highways of London the odour of Continental ghettoes, and bearing in their eyes, through all the shrewdness of their glances, the eternal mysticism of the Orient, where God was born. Hawkers and pedlars, tailors and cigarmakers, cobblers and furriers, glaziers and cap-makers – this was in sum their life: to pray much and to work long.' Flora Tristan, in her *London Journal*, comments on the significance of the used-clothes trades in the East End: 'Oh, the sight of the thousands of old worn-out shoes, the rags and the rubbish and all of it making up such an important branch of commerce gives a truer idea of the destitution of the monster city than all the findings and reports that could be published. It makes one shudder.'

There was intense competition, sometimes resolved by violence, and high seasonal and trade-cycle unemployment. The Whitechapel Road provided an open-air

SOME LIVES!

hiring hall for clothing workers, known as the 'chazer mark' (pig market), an exact parallel to the indignities that dockworkers suffered in the east of the borough. In his *History of a Sweater*, Wilchinski evokes the desperation of hungry men: 'Many of them, like myself, "greeners" [newcomers], willing to work at anything that would bring them the scantiest means of existence; some married and with families and all with that enquiring, beseeching look, that half-starved, helpless, hopeless beings must of necessity possess.' It was the same rough-and-tumble world from which the first Jewish heavyweight boxing champion Daniel Mendoza emerged, a pioneer for his co-religionists, an originator of the East End's pugilistic tradition and author of a boxing textbook which advocates skill and dexterity over brawn. When his old home in Bethnal Green's Paradise Row was dedicated in 1978, bent-nosed, spruce champions of all weights paid tribute before moving on to a civic reception at the York Hall.

At the end of the nineteenth century, the still relatively small Jewish community was swollen by a substantial wave of immigration of Jewish proletarians from Russia and Poland. Under Nicolas I they had been strictly compressed and confined into the Pale of Settlement where they were excluded from secular education and public employment in modernising industries and shovelled instead into petty and insecure occupations, living on the verge of subsistence as pedlars, carters, cigarette-makers, etc. Already on the margin of life and herded into *shtetls*, they were then oppressed by a series of anti-Semitic ukases which William Fishman has described as 'the worst persecution of Jews prior to the Nazi Holocaust'. When they sought to escape from the Baltic and German ports, London was often the first refuge, although for many it was only a stopping point on the journey to Liverpool and thence the United States. Between 1881 and 1905, a million Jews left Russia and Poland, 100,000 coming to Britain, mostly through the London docks.

184

What the immigrants found in the East End was, as always, less than paradise. Aaron Liebermann, a libertarian of the left who had left Russia pursued by the police, wrote: 'In the narrow crooked streets of Whitechapel, in the smelly and dirty holes and corners of the workshops, working 14–16 hours a day for a paltry starvation wage, *here* have the Jewish workers of Russia, Poland and Germany found their better life?' These 'greeners' or newcomers were a distinct embarrassment to the Anglo-Jewish establishment. Their religious habits offended the rabbinate, their efforts to build trade unionism distressed the master tailors, and their sheer numbers, 'foreignness' and lack of education worried the *Jewish Chronicle*. They were also attacked with specific anti-Semitism, often masquerading as a more disinterested 'anti-alienism'. This ranged from abuse, beard-tweaking and desecration to a series of anti-immigration laws passed by 1908 and the foundation in Stepney of the British Brothers League, the first British fascist organisation. In 1898, one-third of Stepney councillors were publicans elected on an anti-Jew, pro-booze ticket.

The Whitechapel settlement was not a formal ghetto of the sort to which the Jews had been legally confined in many European cities, and in this respect it was an emancipation. But Jews were still denied many civil liberties because of their religious beliefs and excluded from many Christian-only trades, charities and educational establishments. The establishment of the Jews' Free School, the John Cass Foundation, the London Jewish Hospital and the numerous other Jewish charities was as much a response to discrimination as an effort at separatism. But as pressure was further whipped up on the 'Alien Question', the Jewish immigration, still predominantly Yiddish-speaking and wearing wide-brimmed hat, beard unshaven and corner of hair uncut, turned inward to the euphoria of Orthodox worship and noisy self-expression in the neighbourhood corner synagogues called *steibels*: then, as now, fundamentalism was one response to oppression. As with the French, the first phase of immigrants were 'more Russian than the Russians' and found great strength and identity from religious observance and ritual.

But in the East End 'the influx' was disconcerting to the authorities. It was noted that the high level of immigration from East Europe coincided with large-scale emigration to North America. Racism and eugenism were quick to surface, propelled by meanness (the St George's in the East Vestry requesting immigration control 'to prevent this country becoming the dust heap of every continental nation') or through explicit imperialist prejudice, as articulated by Captain Colomb, a Victorian Enoch Powell who stated: 'I object to England, with its overcrowded population and small area, being made a human ashpit for the refuse population of the world.' As usual, hygiene was cited, despite the fact that the Jews observed ritual bathing and had in fact established four of their own baths in the East End for this purpose. The Reverend J. C. Billing told the House of Commons Committee on Emigration of 'half-starved miserable Jewish children in the streets, picking up garbage from the gutters and bearing all the traces of disease'. And the veteran anti-alien campaigner Arnold White even exhibited a selection of destitute 'greeners' (who in fact were established immigrants bribed to dress the part by the promise of travel grants).

Respectable established Anglo-Jewish society remained embarrassed by its poverty-stricken co-religionists. Sebag Montefiore put the dilemma frankly: 'While I cannot bring myself to refuse our free shores to persecuted foreigners, I would do all in my power to dissuade those foreigners from coming to our shores.' The Anglo-Jewish establishment did its best to discourage departure from East Europe and arranged dispersal from the East End on arrival. Prejudice was widespread in the sensational press, echoed uncritically in the local newspapers, and even found its way into socialist newspapers like Hyndman's xenophobic *Justice* which carried the editor's anti-Semitic promise to 'reveal the Jew influence in our Cabinets and our most prosperous journals'.

But, shunted by prejudice out of the industrial mainstream and hovering somewhere between poverty and destitution, the only answer was the sweated trades, either at home or in the grim workshops. One was at least with co-religionists, often 'landsmen', people from the same village of origin. Then there was the short-term credit of the pawnbroker, gambling – that staple compensation of the immigrant – and the charities. 'La Soupe' of the Huguenots was reborn as the 'Soup Kitchen' for the Jewish poor, opened by the Chief Rabbi in 1888 in Brune Street, Spitalfields.

But there was an organised resistance to these narrow options which contained an antidote to the fatalistic motto of the Yiddish immigrant, 'Schwer und bitter is dos Leben'. It came initially from politicised refugees from tsardom, men like Aaron Liebermann who had been a member of the anti-tsarist revolutionary left and a peer of Kropotkin and Zasulich, who in 1896 brought together a band of working men from the sweatshops to a meeting in Gun Street to form the first-ever Hebrew socialist union and issue a manifesto aimed primarily at the Jews of Eastern Europe. This group was short-lived, but one of those influenced by it, the poet Morris Vinchevsky, with his friend Rabbinowitz went on to found the first socialist newspaper in Yiddish, the *Poilische Yidl* (the 'Little Polish Jew'), published at 137 Commercial Street, E1, and aiming to 'instruct and support our brothers who know little or nothing of other languages; to help "greeners" who have recently arrived and are seeking work; to give its men and women some insight into world affairs'. As well as pungent and humorous about the exigencies of immigrant life, it was atheistic and had a clear socialist outlook. 'What good is talk when Jewish workers are complaisant and smug and nothing perturbs them? . . . What one cannot or is afraid to do alone, can be done

187

by a host, by a united workers' party.' *Freedom*, the newspaper of William Morris's Commonwealth League, commented approvingly: 'Our Jewish comrades are not only socialist propagandists. They are systematically occupied in organising trade societies to combat the sweated system, raise the rates of wages to subsistence level . . . and communicate the real state of affairs in the London labour market to their brethren abroad.'

The Little Polish Jew's successor was the *Arbeter Fraint* (the 'Worker's Friend'). *Arbeter Fraint* was open 'to all radicals, social democrats, collectivists, communists and anarchists' and edited by the remarkable German goy Rudolph Rocker, who had taught himself Yiddish. The *Arbeter Fraint* in turn built and opened an educational club in Berners Street and then, by mutual aid, the famous Jubilee Street anarchist club which was opened in 1906 by Prince Peter Kropotkin. The club played an important role in the social and intellectual development of all East Enders, with two auditoria, one with a gallery for 800, attached libraries, reading rooms and classroom accommodation. The anarchist club was irreligious and for sexual equality, organising cheap food and drink, balls and benefits, chess, children's Sunday school and excursions to Epping Forest and the British Museum. Above all, it was a place of learning where Morris and Shaw were listened to by tailors and shoe- and cabinet-makers hungry for ideas. Rocker spoke one week on Shakespeare and the next on the significance of Beethoven's Ninth. When I was taken by Bill Fishman to a 1974 Toynbee Hall memorial meeting for Rocker, addressed among others by his son Fermin, there was among the audience, which included some well-heeled businessmen, the same respect, almost reverence for matters of the intellect. 'We anarchists are very tolerant,' they used to say. 'All workers are our comrades. All ideas are our servants.'

From this headquarters, Rocker led two strikes of

great importance for the East End clothing industry: the 1906 strike which was defeated by the master tailors, who, however, conceded the abolition of piecework, a ten-and-a-half-hour working day and the right for trade unions to collect subs. The *Jewish Chronicle* poured lofty scorn on the strikers: it could rebound little to the credit of the East End that crowds of Jewish young men and women, conspicuously more or less new arrivals in the country, should 'invade the westward thoroughfares, flaunting gaudy banners inscribed with revolutionary texts, and affrighting the decorous silence of a London Sunday with a blatant blare of brass'. The Jewish unions, who had lost the 1906 strike through the transfer of work out of London, were ready, as part of a larger wave of syndicalist strikes, to try again in 1912, and this time there was unity with dockers and seamen in London and Liverpool. At a meeting of the united Jewish clothing unions, with over 11,000 present at the Mile End Assembly Rooms, Blythe of the West End Society of Tailors warned that 'trade would come down to the East End to be finished, and the tailors in East London must decline to finish that work or become blacklegs'. After a speech in Yiddish by Rocker, the East Enders voted unanimously for supporting their West End colleagues, and within two days 13,000 immigrant tailors walked out of their workshops.

The *East London Observer*, even more conservative then than it is now, observed sardonically that this 'Gilbertian charade of a really stupid strike' will 'present itself as a mild joke'. But the strike committees were well organised with subcommittees dealing with strategy, funds and negotiation and a drive for strike finance which involved levies, collections, theatre benefits and temporary canteens. *Arbeter Fraint* produced a four-page daily with strike news. There were joint demonstrations on the Mile End waste between tailors and dockers who were preparing for their next great strike. Although drained and exhausted, when the bosses offered a compromise the strikers held out for their last and most important demand, the closed union shop. And the employers, their seasonal trade in ruins, conceded. No more could the Jewish immigrants be associated with strike-breaking. And in support of the docks strike, 300 children from the Poplar area, reduced to 'a terribly undernourished state, barefoot and in rags', were taken into Jewish homes in Whitechapel. The cut-throatism endemic in the ghetto had been turned into its inverse: trade union solidarity.

The First World War devastated this moment which, despite its profound impression on East End culture, was largely extinct as an organised political force by 1920. After the success of the Russian Revolution, many East End socialists returned to the Soviet Union, where they were to meet their deaths at the hands of Stalinism. The Balfour Declaration of 1917 began the long process by which Zionism, hitherto a minority tradition, began to take its toll on Jewish radicalism, until, after the Holocaust, it was to become a major and increasingly reactionary force within the Jewish community.

Simon Blumenfeld's 1930s East End novel *Jew Boy*, for instance, is about a Whitechapel tailor who is keenly aware of anti-Semitism: 'Our own proletarian flesh and blood. Why should they hate us so? What have we done to them? We eat, sleep, drink, work like they do; yet that hatred is always underneath, ready at any moment to flare up in that bitter gibe: JEW! JEW! BLOODY JEW! The priests and parsons and Imperialists had done their work well.' But experience in the workshop and factories had taught him how little nationalism is worth. Arguing with a pretentious middle-class poet, the hero states, 'I haven't the faintest desire to claim Palestine as my own. I believe that wherever a man lives and does useful work and brings up his children, is his country. As a worker, I won't be any better off in Palestine, maybe worse. I don't see why I should change one set of exploiters for another because they happen to be Jewish.'

As the great historian of this period, William Fishman, himself Stepney-born and a principal in Further Education in Tower Hamlets, argues, the Education Acts did much to bring Jewish children into the mainstream of English education. The Royal Commission on Alien Immigration, for example, heard the headmaster of the Deal Street Board School confirm that in his school 'practically the whole of these children are of foreign parentage. Notwithstanding this fact, the lads have become thoroughly English. They have acquired our language. They take a keen and intelligent interest in all that concerns the welfare of our country.'

But assimilation and educational, cultural and business success did not protect against the anti-Semitism which was still widespread in British society. Not only did the British governments of the 1930s strive to keep on good terms with Hitler, but they were ill-disposed to grant visas to German refugees from Nazism who were not themselves well-off. By April 1934, just under 3,000 German Jews had managed to find refuge in Britain, compared with 30,000 in France. Specific pressure from the British Medical Association resulted in the admission of a sizeable group of Jewish doctors. When war broke out, some 50,000 German and Austrian refugees and 6,000 Czechs were afforded refuge, of whom 10,000 were children. And in 1940, 11,000 of the refugees, despite their willingness to volunteer to fight against Nazism, were rounded up and interned.

And Jewish religious orthodoxy was not driven away by a few satires in *Arbeter Fraint*. Yet the radicalism of the East End Jews fed into the East London Communist Party, particularly in Stepney where the CP played an important role in the movement against Mosley, in wartime direct action and the postwar housing and squatting movements. The tradition of supporting strikes remains intact and strong in the East End, even when those strikes are predominantly defensive as they have been in the 1970s and 1980s.

The children of the ghetto pioneers are long gone; I meet their grandchildren now, film directors and professors, teachers and solicitors, whose parents came from the sweatshops in the Mile End Road and the furniture workshops of Bethnal Green. The exit routes are well marked: the 'North West Passage', first to Hackney and Tottenham, thence to Hampstead Garden Suburb and Hendon, or east to Ilford and Woodford, those suburban supporters of the status quo. Many migrated to the USA, returning in raincoats and loud tweeds to make obeisance to Blooms' surly waiters. Those left behind are an elderly population of couples, widows, sisters, marooned by history and becalmed by illness. But still larger than life, the women precisely made up with brittle hair and curly lipstick, the men neat, grey and somehow shrunk. Their self-deprecating stoicism sometimes bursts into wonderful neuroticism: 'Oh, my God, I'm a goner. Whatcha going to do, Doc?' In claustrophobic council houses piled high with objects, belongings, souvenirs which have become familiar hells.

There was a strong Jewish flavour to general practice in the East End. When I first worked in Bethnal Green, the trio of Harry Hyams, Freddy Somers and Mike Leibson, each with his own shopfront surgery, divided the High Street. Although some Jewish doctors were refugees – Somers was said to have walked for a week without food to escape a Polish concentration camp – several were born in Whitechapel and Stepney and had managed to get into the London Hospital in the days when anti-Semitism was still common in medicine. Sam Smith, the Bow GP, recalls being mysteriously unable to get a match with the Rugby Club, 'so I joined the Boxing Club instead and delighted in knocking every anti-Semite out of the ring': a very Stepney reaction. Smith, who had been called before the Medical School dean for supporting the strikers in Poplar in 1926, was a medical officer after the relief of Buchenwald and, for many years, a stalwart communist. His method of teaching medicine was very much the tricks of the trade; dog Latin cough bottles, the tricks to spot a back-pain malingerer, ways of distracting kids in pain, and oblique methods of fishing diagnostically. Leibson would simply draw on his decades of local knowledge: after my long clinical summaries of conflicting findings, he would pause and then snort, 'Well, he's been a silly bugger since that business with Sybil.' Smith had perfected a patriarchal bluffness: 'Look, you know I'm blunt. I don't have the energy to lose my temper with you. You need to sort yourself out instead of whingeing to me.' A patter that was a banter delivered with knowing quick glances and strokes of his goatee: 'Away with you,' he would rasp and indicate the door with his warm walnut eyes. They must have loved him to let him get away with it.

A major source of immigration were the Irish, who have been part of the East End since the sixteenth century. Often arriving with little more than their clothes, they worked in the most degrading of conditions in the docks, the wharves and the riverside industries. Irish women went into service and street-selling. Both sexes were habitually denounced for loose morals and beggary as well as 'Papism', the religious rationale for much anti-Irish prejudice. Even when Liverpool and Manchester became more popular destinations for the Irish forced from their country by English landlordism and Irish commercial backwardness, East London retained a number of Catholic churches including the vast St Joseph's basilica in Poplar, schools and many social clubs. Irish names have been prominent in municipal politics. The role of the priesthood in raising East End Irish educational standards has been considerable, but being devout on Sunday has not stopped East End Irish being active republicans and unionists. East London was a centre of both Anti-Internment and Troops Out movements in the 1970s. A meeting calling for the release of the Birmingham Six will still bring 800 or 900 mainly Irish workers to Hackney Town Hall. For to see the East London Irish as supplying mainly brawn is to miss their contribution to the organisation of the Labour and trade union movement and the tenacity of their political loyalty. It is also to miss, in the mists of Catholicism, the importance of a London republican presence.

Irish immigration increased again in line with the booms in the London financial and construction sectors in the mid 1980s, sucking in another generation of Southern Irish in search of work. Once again, London's barn-like pubs in Holloway, Cricklewood, Camden and Hammersmith filled with young people looking for a shout and a stout with a shamrock on it, but more likely to be singing along to the Pogues than McAlpine's Fusiliers. The Irish pubs of the East End still remain, in their quiet way, social centres with their ambitious Sunday drinking, sharp-twanged volunteer singers and cheerful children. St Patrick's Night in the 'White Hart' in Stoke Newington High Street could be in Kerry: couples waltzing, sweepstake collections, gentlemen in trilbies talking sadly of the fate of their horses. And at the bar, a Cork mohican with Miles Davis T-shirt buying eight pints of Guinness. In a way, this is the heart of modern proletarian London. As the Pogues sing in 'London, You're a Lady': 'Your architects were madmen, your builders sane but drunk. And among your faded jewels shine acid house and punk.'

In addition, a Chinese community was established on the Limehouse dockside as early as 1880. The original Chinese East Enders were seamen and cooks from the boats of the East India Company, who set up shops and restaurants catering mostly for fellow Chinese in Limehouse, the original Chinatown. It was a self-enclosed community, although much abused as criminal and drug-dealing. The area was decimated during the Blitz, and the scale of the settlement can now only be understood by looking at the Chinese graves in the East London Cemetery in Grange Road, E13. The original colony was swelled in the late nineteenth century by seamen paid off due to the sale or scrapping of their ships. The shipowners had a legal obligation to repatriate their ex-employees but, anxious to avoid the expense, did not look too hard. The seamen from Shanghai settled in the Pennyfields area, while those from Canton preferred Gill Street and Limehouse Causeway. (It is in Gill Street that Sax Rohmer's invention Fu-Manchu, the Asiatic master criminal, is first sighted.) By 1915 the area was largely Chinese, with lodging houses, clubs and a Christian mission. The physical structure of this old Chinatown was destroyed in the Blitz, although the rebuilding provided accommodation for some of the principal restaurants round whose spinning tables East End families have enjoyed eating out for generations.

There was, especially in Limehouse, a good deal of intermarriage: it is not uncommon to meet Chinese-Jewish families, or Anglo-Chinese waitresses in restaurants. Limehouse was also a resettlement point of Vietnamese refugees in the 1980s. This wave of immigration, although quite small, was organised in a more systematic way with transit centres and an attempt to disperse migrants to different destinations in Britain, including Glasgow and Teesside. In fact, the Vietnamese arrivals, usually from fishing or peasant families in the ports of North Vietnam, had little in common with the existing Chinese community although some spoke Cantonese. But, unlike the Chinese, they came *en masse* and *en famille* and are bringing up young families in the old tenements.

Chinese culture was not as pulverised by colonialism as African or Asian: Cantonese is the most widely spoken language in the world, and Chinese culture was both ancient and advanced. London-Chinese identity is self-confident but not aggressive. Indeed, the traditional self-sufficiency of the Chinese community is often taken up by the authorities as an excuse for withholding deserved resources. As the Chinese Information and Advice Centre commented, 'The Chinese community is waking up, almost too late, to place our demands on a welfare state which is withering away.'

Those leaving Vietnam have arrived in London not only after a hazardous journey but long periods in the internment camps in Sek Kong or Thai Ah Chaue in Hong Kong, waiting endlessly in unhygienic hammocks and on hard benches for their processing. The wealthy Hong Kong financiers may have access protected and the money to buy into the LDDC area, but the boat people arrive visibly and mentally exhausted by their terrifying journey and often carrying the scars of long-term incarceration and uncertainty. The difficult transition from pyjamas, siestas and an outdoor life to the dark, dank concrete council estates of East London undoubtedly contributes to the high incidence of stress-related illness. The imagined 'American Dream' of highly paid job, colour TV and big car is still as far away as ever. Many Vietnamese men work in low-paid unskilled jobs, and Vietnamese food has made relatively little inroad. The Vietnamese, like other recent immigrants, often acquire the worst eating habits of the indigenous society: in particular sugar, scarce in Vietnam, is eaten in excess. Lamb, milk and dairy products will probably be unfamiliar too. And although the Vietnamese pride themselves on stoicism, the sheer drama of their journey to the West (nearly 5,000 were shipwrecked and rescued by British ships) and the continuing desperation of those 50,000 compatriots herded into transit camps in Hong Kong, must weigh heavily. As you arrange for a wheelchair or support a naturalisation affidavit, you sense the pain of migration for people whose English is rudimentary, who have no power and only a weak community and who look at authority, even the doctor, with imploring, uncomprehending faces.

Other twentieth-century migrants were African, seamen from Somalia, Ethiopia and East Africa who settled in the old Cable Street area of Stepney, joined by Mediterranean peoples from North Italy, Greece, Cyprus and Malta. Twelve thousand Gibraltarians were evacuated in 1940 and several thousand ex-naval dockyard workers from Malta came in 1950. So postwar Cable Street, demolished in the 1960s, gained its reputation for raucous red-light partying behind some fairly nondescript curtained cafés wedged between bomb-damaged rubble.

After the Second World War, when the British workforce was cut by war deaths and emigration to the 'White Commonwealth', immigration law was specifically altered by the 1948 Nationalities Act to encourage immigration from what were still the colonies of the West Indies, India and Pakistan. Being a British colony meant exactly that: exclusion from the good land by the vast London-owned plantations and estates, social relations still diffused with the traditions of slavery, political servility, brutal policing and rudimentary schooling. So when Jamaican men, many of them ex-armed forces, took a chance on the *Emperor Windrush* single voyage to the Pool of London, it was a desperate gamble and an act of some courage. The men were not sure if they would be allowed to disembark, where they would live (few had relatives or contacts), or what work they could do. There was no regular boat service (the *Windrush* was returning from Australia) to get them back and, on arrival, they were accommodated at the last moment in a Clapham deep bomb shelter. Recalls Baron Baker, one of the Jamaican Pilgrim Fathers who pioneered the Brixton settlement: 'To find another coloured man I had to go Aldgate East.' Stepping ashore at Tilbury with snow-white cuffs, correspondent shoes, painted ties and innocent smiles, the Jamaicans were entering a social minefield where the colour bar was widespread, physical attack common and prejudice deep-rooted. Old patients, now grizzled grandfathers and mothers, recall those days in East London with a mixture of warmth and terror.

In fact, as Hogarth's paintings show so clearly, there is a long-standing Black London. Although slavery was always illegal, it is probable that the first black settlers in the East End were freed slaves who came to London as personal servants of the sea captains who lived in fine houses near the river. There is evidence that at least two well-known Wapping inns ran slave markets. But it is also the paradoxical case that many freed blacks lived independently and were held in some respect in particular dockside trades. The black population in London in the eighteenth century was thus predominantly male and in the east of London. It was based on sea trades but included musicians, entertainers and servants. Slaves were certainly still bought and sold as late as the 1760s. A newspaper advertisement of the period runs: 'Run away from his master about a Fortnight since, a lusty Negroe boy, about 18 years of Age, full of pock holes: had a silver collar about his neck engrav'd Capt. Thos. Mitchel's Negroe, living in Griffith St in Shadwell.' Those not in livery were in rags. Slavery in Britain was only formally abolished by a ruling in 1772 which forbade a slave who deserted his master from being recaptured by force to be sold abroad. But freed slaves and the poor of East London both played an important part in the Abolition Movement which succeeded in stopping the 'triangular' slave trade in 1807, by which time its importance to imperialism had greatly diminished anyway. It was only with the new economic links with the Caribbean and West Africa, through the fruit trade lines in the late nineteenth century, that distinctive black port communities emerged in Cable Street and Canning Town in the East End, in Cardiff's Tiger Bay and in Liverpool 8.

Contrary to popular belief, Asians have been in the East End for a long time, because the East India Company, whose monopoly was established in 1600, had its docks and its administrative headquarters in Poplar and the City. Asians were first seen as seamen, known as 'lascars', sometimes deliberately stranded in port by their company, and also as 'ayahs', nurses to white colonial families, who were also often evicted and left to fend for themselves in London. If, as some contemporary accounts suggest, they were often reduced to beggary, this destitution was simply due to being dumped or deserting ship to escape cruel treatment on board. The relationship with Sylhet in the flood delta of the Bay of Bengal was forged through the East India Company who, through the military conquests of Clive, succeeded the Mughal Empire in utilising the area for the extraction of lime and collecting of land rents. As Sir William Hunter put it, in his *Annals of Rural Bengal*, 'Bengal was regarded by the British public in the light of a vast warehouse, in which a number of adventurous Englishmen carried on business with great profit on an enormous scale. That a numerous native population existed they were aware of, but this they considered an accidental circumstance.' Before imperial conquest, its saltpetre and silks had been important exported manufactures.

The East India Company moved from trade to conquest, and Bengal effectively became a company province where the British had the right to raise and collect taxes. Although the nabobs attained enormous personal wealth which was used to bankroll the industrial revolution, the profits of empire did very little for the working men and women of East London, locked outside the treasure rooms. Natives of India were in turn planted all over the British Empire as labourers and petty administrators, so that Indians worked the plantations of Burma and the mines of South Africa, constructed the East India railway and fought the wars to extend the frontiers of empire.

Sylhet, in North Bengal, was a land of elephants, tigers, seamen, cooks and adventurers. It had an indigenous fine textile industry which was effectively dismantled by the Company, who then proceeded to import British manufactured cloth. It was only in the mid-nineteenth century that tea was discovered, growing wild. But by the end of the century, tea-planting and the shipping lines which exported it to London had become the major industry. The cultivators were, paradoxically, peasants possessing their own land but with a very low income. Relatively well-off men went to sea by choice rather than as a last resort. It is also said that the inhabitants of Sylhet, due to Arab blood, are particularly bold, inquiring and fond of travel. Officially, Sylheti men could only crew the shipping routes east of the Cape of Good Hope. But this rule was relaxed for crews in Europe-bound steam packets by the mid-nineteenth century. Access to a job on board was via a shipping broker who also provided accommodation while waiting for a berth, and extended credit. Both he and the ship's bosun would need a sizeable bribe, but this system consolidated the close relationship with the sailors of Sylhet and certain of the British shipping lines.

It was said that the maritime division of labour was for the Muslims to go in the boiler, Hindus on the decks and Christian converts in the saloon. Sylhetis had something of a monopoly on stokers' jobs for the steam boats carrying tea and jute out of Calcutta. They appealed to the owners because their wages were very low, they worked hard and didn't drink. It was only as late as 1941 that the system of bribery to get a shipboard job was replaced by an open muster where seamen were selected on a more impartial basis. Once on board, life must have been extremely grim: long shifts and the hardest work, oiling and greasing in the engine rooms, firing and cleaning the boilers and cutting the coal slabs, paid under 'lascar articles' about a twentieth of the British crew wages, being shouted orders by the ships' officers in 'lascari bat' and cooking their own meals on deck from dried fish and meat and rice and dhal. By 1939, 50,000 out of 190,000 sailors in the British Merchant Marine were under lascar articles. Pitched into the wartime North Atlantic and Baltic runs, the Bengali boilermen were the first to be hit by torpedo attack. If not killed instantly, they were likely to drown in oily water or slip off the life-raft rat ropes into the freezing depths. Yet only a few of the names of these young men who served so bravely in a war which had little to do with them are even recorded.

A few Sylheti pioneers had established hostels and coffee-houses in both the East End and the West End of London before the Second War. They were entirely legal, being citizens of the empire who had only journeyed from the second city of the empire, Calcutta, to the first. But after the war, more men sought their fortune in London. The clothing trade was still predominantly Jewish but the ex-seamen found jobs out of sight in the luxury hotels as boilermen, porters and spud bashers. There were the rudiments of community; the East London Mosque in Commercial Street, a backyard halal slaughterhouse, the first Muslim undertaker near Cable Street, and the first of the 'Indian' restaurants catering for a white, often ex-colonial, clientele who could polish up their Anglo-Hindustani on the waiters. But the London Sylheti community was as small as 300 by the early 1950s. The historian Caroline Adams, however, has established its political importance in sustaining the exiles who were to lead the successful struggle for the independence of Bangladesh from Pakistani rule. Although Bengalis went to work in the cotton mills of Oldham, the steel mills of Sheffield and Scunthorpe and the foundries of Leeds and Smethwick, the East End settlement, perhaps 5,000 strong by 1962, retained a clear pre-eminence, and by 1985 a fifth of all Britain's 100,000 Bangladeshis were in Tower Hamlets.

The community is young and fertile now that, after long delays, families are united in Britain and East End-born Bangladeshis are themselves becoming parents. But the economic boom which created the full employment that sucked immigrants into Britain in the 1950s and early 1960s is long gone, with fatal effects on many of the heavy industries in which the Bangladeshis had previously been employed. In particular, the character of the textile trade has been transformed by the collapse of manufacture in Britain in the face of competition from South-East Asian manufacturers. As the last major migrant group to East London, coming from one of the poorest parts of the world, the Bangladeshis have a particularly tough time. While single men could, just, put up with multiple occupation, this is intolerable when family arrives. Earlier Pakistani and West Indian migrants, when barred from access to council housing lists, were sometimes able to save up to purchase housing, but house price inflation ruled this out for the Bangladeshis who were instead concentrated in the oldest and worst accommodation in the east.

There has been little new council building since the early 1970s and much of what exists is in poor repair or of unsuitable size. So the East End immigrants have once again become the subject of a Parliamentary Commission which concluded that the government was 'failing in its housing responsibilities in the area, which was causing tremendous damage not just to the Bangladeshis but to all inhabitants of Tower Hamlets through reduced availability of council accommodation'. It went on: 'It is hard to imagine anything more damaging to racial harmony in Tower Hamlets than competition between different communities for increasingly scarce housing.'

Some of the housing in which the Bangladeshis lived was atrocious and one needs no more sophisticated instrument than a pair of eyes to measure this. The housing around Brick Lane was the oldest and the most decrepit in the borough, often with outside toilets, no bathrooms, and leaking roofs and gutters. There was little council housing visible, although there were several tenements of the sort which may have been model dwellings a hundred years ago but which were now decayed and depressing. Although hardened to bad housing, I can still remember the shock of visiting the shared home of six male Bangladeshi clothing workers in Hanbury Street in the early 1970s. It was summer and the forecourt stank of food rubbish dumped from the restaurants and uncollected by the borough. The flat was dark and bare, a night shelter

more than a home, all its windows barred with hardboard. There was an old-fashioned sink and a tap with
cold water only. The young man with abdominal pain
(which turned out to be appendicitis) was doubled up
in agony on a shared mattress on the floor. None of
the men was registered with a doctor or knew where
the hospital was. In this bleak room they had lived
a sealed-off life, self-sufficient in the extremity of its
poverty, grateful to be exploited by co-religionists,
hope for the future as barred as the windows.

The dispersal of the Brick Lane enclave at first worsened the situation. When wives, often much younger,
and the children conceived on holiday visits joined the
father, the eventual housing offer was to the most
unpopular estates where the new arrivals would often
be the first Bengali family in the block. Isolation from
shops, mosque and Sylheti speakers would be immediately compounded by physical attack. Nearly eighty
years ago, in the anti-alien rioting, a broken window
was called 'the sincerest form of flattery'. Window-
breaking is a simple but effective form of harassment.
It is easy to execute and repeat, runs low risk to the
assailant and usually ends in the attacked tenant having
to barricade the window with chicken wire and boards
producing permanent darkness inside. In the
mid-1970s, such arrangements were universally
required by Bangladeshi families rehoused in East
Bethnal Green. And window-breaking is arguably less
serious than the arson, sari-ripping and public attacks
which were also commonplace and at the time given
little attention by the police. At night, there was a
virtual curfew and by day the people moved about only
in groups: to the doctor *en famille* even if only one
child was ill. The women went to work in the clothing
factories in groups of ten. A 'Warning Dog Patrol'
sign went up outside the Brick Lane mosque, pregnant
women walked *en masse* to antenatal clinics, minicabs
specialised in taking people to work and school even if
the journey was only 400 yards, and Asian schoolkids

had to be let out early so that they would get home unmolested.

The medical results were frequently diffuse somatic symptoms which were almost always secondary to depression. During the height of the racist agitation in 1976, I was perpetually being called out by young children who should have been in school to visit their mothers having the vapours on elongated home-made beds behind barred windows and doors with a cluster of locks and bolts. And the men had an alarmingly high incidence of heart attacks, stomach ulcers and diabetes. Having made a transition from rural tranquillity to the heart of one of the biggest metropolises in the world, they had to bring up and provide for their large young families isolated from relatives and locked indoors for their own safety. And frequently they were suffering from infectious respiratory diseases, skin infections and fevers which became almost endemic in their over-crowded and poorly heated homes. 'Pain all over' was a fairly precise transcription of what they must have been feeling.

Some of the housing transfers were almost ludicrous. Coventry Cross is a spur of 1930s housing completely cut off from shops by the Blackwall Tunnel Approach motorway. No one wants to live there apart from tran-sitory squatters usually involved in petty crime or drug-dealing. Dogs run wild in packs, burnt-out cars line the entrance. The place is less welcoming than most prisons and it's about as far away from Brick Lane as you can get within the borough. To billet Asian families there without support is to condemn them before they have started to becoming the inevitable scapegoat of the resentful residents themselves awaiting rehousing. Bengali families transferred to Teviot Estate in Poplar were quite literally burnt out. At the height of National Front activity there was more violence than anything undertaken by the Mosleyites and the smell of pogrom was in the air.

Eventually the racist tide was turned, by physical

defence of both Brick Lane and the isolated families, by a propaganda offensive against the NF by the Anti-Nazi League and Rock Against Racism, and by a newfound confidence in the Asians of Tower Hamlets themselves. As Ken Leech has written: 'The emergence of a new Bengali radicalism is the most hopeful and most encouraging aspect of the whole period. . . . The ghetto has produced not despair and resignation but anger and organised revolt.' For the achievement of the Asians in finding their own feet and, in the process, a new identity is no less formidable than the earlier Jewish migration which took from Rudolph Rocker to Arnold Wesker's communist Auntie Sadie, or from the 1889 dock strike to the battle of Cable Street – that is, three full generations – to find their Cockney footing. We do not yet know the identity of the Bengali Bronowski, the Asian Mikardo, or the Sylheti Wesker, but they will assuredly come. And the lads in their bomber jackets and the young women in their saris, trousers and stilettos will make yet another generation of Cockneys.

There is, however, no room for complacency: the next recession could once again tempt people towards racialist explanations. Caroline Adams's recent interviews with some pioneers of the older generation reflect their concern about the heartlessness of Britain in the 1990s. Says Abdul Wahab: 'England used to be much better than it is now. In those days people were very, very friendly but now Bengali people get attacked.' Mr Ayyar Ullah says: 'The roads are better but the people are worse.' Syed Rasul remembers: 'Those times were very different – not much money, but you got everything and you were very happy.' Haji Shirajul Islam suggests: 'Things have changed here. In the old days people were just the same as our people, we were all one. All they want to do now is bashing and stabbing and beating.' And this reflects, sadly, not their sentimentality but the increasingly brutal and careless place we have allowed Britain to become.

So East London, like all inner London, has been

shaped, made what it is, by immigration, much of it from the old colonies of the British Empire. In some way it is like imperialism rolled into reverse gear; one of the migrant organisations' most succinct slogans is 'We are here because you were there'.

So if the city could talk, or when it finds its voice, the once-immigrants, now East Enders, will have some fine tales to tell. And when London's radical history is written, we may see in the immigrants' contribution to the industrial roll of honour at Woolfs Rubber, Perivale Gutermann and Grunwicks, in the mass funerals of the victims of racist attack and police malpractice like Michael Ferreira and Altab Ali, Cherry Groce and Cynthia Jarrett, and in the defiant musical and street cultures a modern equivalent of the values and the struggles of the great days of East End trade unionism in its pioneer pre-bureaucratic time.

CHAPTER 12

DOCKS INTO DOCKLAND

London was a port before it was a city. To the Romans Londinium was a bend in the river, shallow enough to moor the galleys which offloaded the troops and provisions to sustain an army of occupation at the edge of its empire. The first port was 'hithes', moorings cut into the clay of the river bank and strengthened by stakes. As the importance of London as a trading centre grew, the loading and unloading of boats took place in the Pool of London to lighters which would ferry cargo to shore or at quays where ships could moor alongside jetties such as Billingsgate, Puddle Dock and St Mary Overie. The first enclosed wet dock was at Blackwall as part of the East India Company's establishment mentioned by Pepys in 1661. But unloading mainly took place at the 1,400-foot 'Legal Quays' where duty was levied by the Revenue on mounds of imports heaped on the riverside. Despite the addition of the Sufferance Quays (which had, allegedly, only a short-term right to unload but in fact charged more than the legal quays), they were hopelessly inadequate as eighteenth-century London became the largest city in Europe and by far the biggest town in Britain. Seventy per cent of all British sea trade passed through the Port of London and the city's inhabitants relied on the coastal boats for fuel, provisions and food. Despite the extensive network of dry and wet docks in which ships were built and repaired downriver, the upriver facilities for docking and unloading were congested, inefficient and vulnerable to crime.

They were also extremely lucrative for the Corporation of London who had in the twelfth century purchased the sole rights to the use of these quays from Richard Coeur de Lion for £20,000, used to finance the crusades. But by the end of the eighteenth century, a corrupt bedlam prevailed as some 3,500 ocean-going boats and 10,000 vessels in the coastal trade queued at anchor up to six miles downstream awaiting their turn at the quays. The congestion worsened between July and October, when trade winds blew the sugar-, rum- and spice-laden West Indiamen in together. The queuing ships were sitting targets for the organised riverside criminals who were efficient, specialised and often in cahoots with the ships' masters, corrupt revenue officers and complicit watchmen. River pirates would loot unguarded ships; 'heavy horsemen' by day and 'light horsemen' by night. 'Mudlarks', under the pretence of looking for scrap metal, would snatch cargo from boat hatches. And 'scuffle hunters' were adept at concealing stolen goods under their aprons. Because there was little warehousing and goods waited for long periods pending payment of duty, dockside pilfering was universal. Rogues River was costing the companies over £500,000 a year with as much as half of the cargoes vanishing *en route*.

The Scottish pamphleteer and merchant Patrick Colquhoun, affronted by the scale of criminality, in 1800 penned an influential treatise, 'On the Commerce and the Police of the River Thames', which recommended a specialised paramilitary armed guard. This was duly established in Wapping, with ex-watermen and sailors recruited as constables who fought hand to hand with the smugglers and thieves. He also proposed that, in return for some guarantee of employment, the West India Company 'lumpers' would have to consent to wearing only specified clothes and submit to searches on leaving the ships: 'only Stockings and Breeches – no Frocks, Trowsers, Jemmies, Pouches, or Bags'. But these measures would never have succeeded without reform of the wharf system to give greater physical security.

This had been recommended by a parliamentary committee in 1796, but instead of a single, large-scale scheme, individual rival commercial docks were built piecemeal in the then largely uninhabited marshy down-river areas. Although they varied widely in size, from the eventual 245 acres of the Royal Group to the 10-acre St Katherine's Dock, the area covered by the enclosed upriver docks was eventually to be bigger than the City of Venice. Unlike the pattern of municipal docks in Liverpool, all London docks were privately owned. They were built in the face of fierce opposition from both City and traditional trades like lightermen and porters. The first was built in 1802 by the West India Company on the site of the original Blackwall Dock on the Isle of Dogs, then known only for its pasture and its windmills. It set an architectural pattern which was to define social relations in East London. For it was as much a fortified compound as an unloading bay ringed by massive external walls which the architect Jessop promised would 'be very much stronger at the end of a Century when it shall have got in it the ingredient that has given Celebrity to the Cement of the Ancients, which is Time'. Just as it was protected from the Thames tides by a lock system at the entry to the thirty-acre Import Dock and the twenty-four-acre Export Dock, it was protected from the poverty-stricken local inhabitants by almost medieval fortifications of walls and ditches and its own internal police force and military guard, 'each with a good Muskett and Bayonet'. The locks were linked with basins so that vessels could gather on the high tide and be locked through together to the five-storey warehouses which were opened by Pitt with great celebration and a public holiday.

Constructed by Irish and Scottish navvies with the aid of steam power, using 24 million bricks brought into place by Jessop through his own Grand Union Canal, it narrowly beat the London Dock into operation and survived the fears that the 'numerous Classes engaged in a System of Plunderage' might try to burn it down. The new buildings were officially designated licensed bonded warehouses and led to London's subsequent pre-eminence as an entrepot port. Boats were spared the three-mile haul round the island, turn-round time fell from four weeks to four days, and thefts of rum and sugar plummeted.

Other docks followed in swift succession, each with its own speciality. The East India merchants whose tea cutters, being greater in depth, had previously unloaded upriver, constructed a dock near the mouth of the River Lea which, until the opening of the Commercial Road, was reached only by water. And the London Dock, whose architect Alexander went on to design the prisons at Maidstone and Dartmoor, was built at Wapping with a twenty-one-year monopoly on all tobacco, rice, wine and brandy imports not covered by the West India and East India monopolies. It was an advanced design, its ventilated storehouses having a vast cellarage and stone buildings famous for their exposed ammonites. Last in this phase of building came the St Katherine's Dock, driven through by Telford, displacing 11,300 inhabitants in order to take advantage of the ending of the London Dock's monopoly. Later dock developments included facilities for unloading coal and salt at Limehouse Basin, and the only South Bank enclosed dock, the 120-acre complex of the Surrey Commercial Docks at Rotherhithe, completed in 1807 on the old site of the original Howland Dock and specialising in the Baltic softwood trade. Dockmania was subsequent to the Victorian enthusiasm for canal building and eclipsed only by the railway boom.

The nineteenth-century Port of London was still the biggest in the world both in volume of goods and dock area, taking most of the Far Eastern trade, half of the Caribbean and a third of the Baltic, and dealing with vast quantities of dried fruits, wine, tea, grain and wool. And the dockers, often descendants of the labourers who had built the brick structures, were developing their particular communities which, although cut off from the rest of London, were cosmopolitan and familiar with the alien. Seamen from the world's ports jigged in pubs and drank in brothels, the spars and masts pushed between the narrow streets, immigrants stood in orderly lines, and roads were named after Pekin, Havana and Malabar. Until the building of the majestic complex of the Royals between 1855 and 1921, the plan of the docks did not change a lot, although they were ingeniously expanded and adapted. But port industries grew in size and importance, notably refinery and ship repair but also handling and manufacture of chemicals, building aggregates and animal foodstuffs. These had been joined by the 'obnoxious industries' London County Council judged best located outside the boundaries of the city proper: slaughtering, tanning, glue-making and gas manufacture. The superimposition of these and the river-related industries on what had been rural or market gardening hamlets required a massive expansion of residential housing provided by builder-speculators like Cubitt, who bought cheap land and pattern-built estates for rent. So by the end of the nineteenth century, East London, especially the riverside boroughs, was immensely crowded with workers who laboured hard with poor working conditions in all weathers. Job security was very low. With such a large reserve army of labour, anyone making inconvenient demands could be replaced by another willing to grin and bear it. Some work was so casual it might only be for an hour. The port official who hired the thirteen-strong gangs of dockers was called a labour master, with its echoes of the Deep South of America.

The creation of trade unions for manual workers in East London is usually identified with the dock strike

211

of 1889. This was a fiercely fought struggle with mass picketing, solidarity stoppages and 16,000-strong marches into the West End. It broke down the Pale which had thus far separated the Anglo-Irish dock districts from the Spitalfields and Stepney areas of clothing manufacture manned by East European Jews. The Jewish families took in and fed dockers' children for the duration of the dispute. But although the strike succeeded, the work was still arbitrary and back-breaking, exposed to wind and cold, waiting in all hours and conditions for 'call ons' with a high accident rate and in foul working conditions. Yet, through the hands of these men, shoulders calloused with the bruising of planks and inflamed by the humping of casks, went the wealth of empire, from raw plantation sugar, West Indian coffee and rum through to African ivory, carpets from Persia, Virginia tobacco hogsheads which took a gang of men to saw in half, and all the tea in China. A Parliamentary Commission reported on the dockers' working conditions that 'only in the mines are the risks greater'. The shareholders, however, basked 'in the sunshine of their annual ten per cent', a dividend which they could afford to spend on the luxury items of empire.

By the end of the nineteenth century, despite the increase in capacity, the port was once again in financial trouble, squeezed at one side by the competition from its rivals at Bristol and Liverpool and at the other by the growing pressure from the workforce for better pay and conditions. The docks were adequate in size but anarchically administered and still causing too much delay for the faster steam-powered vessels. So, effectively, in 1909 the private docks were nationalised by the acquisition of their assets through the issue of Port of London stock. The newly formed Port of London Authority (PLA) also embarked upon extending the Royal Group with the King George V Dock's sixty-four acres of enclosed water. The PLA levied dues on ships and cargoes entering the river and docks, supplied river services and had conservancy duties associated with navigation, charting and the licensing of lighter-men and watermen. The upriver PLA docks continued to be busy and profit-generating through most of the twentieth century, especially after modernisation and greater investment in the postwar period. The London Docks, however, faced increasing pressure from Tilbury which could handle larger boats. When trade fluctuated, the dock owners lost profit because their overheads were fixed. And decasualisation had put considerable potential in the hands of the unofficial docks shop stewards' committees whose impromptu, unpredictable and highly effective action distressed the ship owners. Air cargo transport was becoming cheaper. In the 1930s, the General Steam and Guinness Boats, the Cunarders and the P & O passenger steamers still safely berthed in the enclosed dock system. But the docks were sliding down the river to the ships instead of the ships sailing up the river to the docks. The Quebec Dock in the Surrey Dock system, opened in 1920, and the floating crane were just two of the innovations which enabled the PLA to reassert London's maritime supremacy. Various forms of mechanisation were introduced: conveyor belts, electric trolleys, forklift trucks and containerisation. The war confirmed the massive industrial potential of the docks and the dockers. Two million tons of provisions were unloaded by London dockers in a secret improvised Scottish port, while in London docks were dried out to build Mulberries, prefabricated concrete caissons. On 6 June 1944, 209 ships with 1,000 barges sailed down the River Thames, the biggest invasion force ever assembled.

Dockers were rewarded after the war with the National Dock Labour Board which supervised working conditions. Forklift and palletisation increased storage capacity, roll-on, roll-off methods (derived from wartime tank-landing craft) increased speed, pneumatic pumps sucked grain into vast silos and wine was hydraulically removed into underground tanks. Most of all, containers, first utilised in the 1920s by the Dublin biscuit manufacturer Jacobs, were introduced, seen by the PLA as a way of bypassing the dock unions since the unit containers could be 'stripped', that is, unpacked by non-union labour at their eventual destination. Increasingly, in the PLA it was the accountants who were able to call the shots. And they realised that their vast acreage so near the commercial centre of London had far greater profit-making capacity as land for office expansion than as a dock which could be displaced to Tilbury. The closure of first the London and St Katherine's docks in 1968–9 raised the question of Docklands' future. For this was not just a strip of real estate along the river but, with the right sort of public planning, a major resource for all of London. Should its future identity be shaped by those who lived in it or those who owned the title deeds? The Abercrombie Plan for the postwar reconstruction of London had called for the riverfront to become an open public amenity with St Katherine's Dock a new public park and concert hall. And the subsequent Travers Morgan Plan offered five options, which included the retention of a substantial shipping function and some imaginative ideas about floating New Towns. But the scale of what was at stake was concealed intellectually from Londoners as effectively as the old dock walls had once cut off the cargoes' secrets from prying eyes. This was the biggest planning opportunity London had had in several centuries and one which would shape the capital's entry into the twenty-first century. Yet hardly anybody knew a debate was on.

The first approach was via the Docklands Joint Committee which linked the five boroughs affected with the Greater London Council, then the strategic planning authority. Although it was slow to gain momentum, this plan was a genuine attempt to deal with London's acute housing needs, arrest industrial decline, improve community health and the poor schooling, and offer further educational facilities in the dockland boroughs.

It is to this interregnum we owe the South Poplar and Barkantine Health Centres, the Cannon Industrial Workshops and the arrival of the first supermarket on the Isle of Dogs. It was a step in a direction which might at last have rewarded the communities which had endured the building, the labouring, the bombing and now the closure of the docks. In the Royals, local people drew up suggestions for the future of the 900-acre dock area which retained a freight role. They are now a series of 'ifs': if the Channel rail route had been centred on Stratford rather than King's Cross, if the PLA had looked properly at non-container traffic, Third World shipping lines and even short-haul sea container traffic, if the disastrous 'Stolport' had not been foisted on to the dock, if the powers that be had given a damn, the Royals could still be a going, employing concern instead of the wasteland they have once again become.

But something more sinister was to replace the loveliness of the ships at night on the still water behind the high dock walls. It arrived in the wake of the electoral victory of Margaret Thatcher in 1979: the London Docklands Development Corporation. The LDDC was the first of the new Conservative Government's prototypes for regenerating the inner cities. Its rationale possessed superficial merit, especially when set against the stagnation of the Callaghan Government's impasse and the slow progress of the Docklands Joint Committee. UDCs were to sweep away inertia, slice through red tape and produce tangible results fast. In the favourite word of the civil servants of the Department of the Environment, they were to be 'single-minded', and not become distracted by petty concerns of planning or social provision. Instead the LDDC has proved a highly secretive engine of corruption, a government-financed estate agent which has done to the Docklands what the Highland Clearances did to the north of Scotland. Its set-up has a startling simplicity. A line was drawn round the perimeter of the riverside area which excluded the residential centres like Canning Town but included the docks and dock buildings themselves, a total area of 150 acres, about half of which was classed as 'derelict', that is to say, unoccupied and ripe for development. Inside this vast zone, the (unelected) LDDC was the sole planning authority and very soon the main landowner, able to purchase vast tracts of land at the artificially low prices that then appertained from the PLA and the boroughs with their annual government grant of £90 million. Having made basic improvements in amenities, little more than the levelling and decontamination of sites under the impetus of the 1970s property boom, it was then able to sell on to speculators at prices which were still attractive.

Not only was the site price artificially low and the environmental work heavily subsidised, but the developers could offset the cost of their building against tax and enjoyed a ten-year rate holiday (during which the local rate would be paid on their behalf by the taxpayer). There was also virtually no control over the style and disposition of new building and, apart from a rudimentary and soon inadequate central road, no planning of development or the mix of business, industry and residence. You could put up an office block in E14 more easily than a garage extension in Henley. It was *laissez-faire* gone mad, with less supervision than the Yukon gold rush. If a porn magazine wanted to buy a patch (Northern Cross, publishers of *Penthouse*, were one of the first corporate purchasers) they could do as they pleased. While nextdoor a Dutch property firm could, pretty much according to architectural whim, erect a street of neo-Jacobean, crypto-Georgian, system-built town houses with gingerbread gutters and wrought-iron balconies. Most developers went for a nominal 'mixed' construction (which meant they hadn't yet worked out what would make the most money). For once land values started to accelerate, then, unhindered by the need for planning permission, they could sell on to another consortium who could redefine the site's use yet again. The London Arena started its career as a badly needed indoor sports stadium with an extensive running track but, several changes of ownership later, became a multipurpose auditorium for incoming spectators. Classically, no one remembered to provide parking.

Docklands land prices were now safely on board the general London and South-East England inflationary spiral which had started with a vengeance in the mid-1980s. This was assisted by the massive PR and advertising campaign which aimed to replace sordid images of dockers and Cockneys with those of executive wind-surfing and loft-living. So in the mid-1980s, when it should have been investing in transport, social and health provision, the LDDC was instead cheerleader of the Lawson 'boom', able to promise land purchasers an investment with a guaranteed annual profit of 20 per cent if they did nothing, sizeable tax savings on whatever they erected and complete freedom to do their own thing. An architectural jumble sale emerged on the Isle of Dogs where the dense pattern of streets and community which has shaped East London was replaced with indiscriminate rows of buildings quite incompatible in height, style and purpose and unlinked by anything except builders' rubble. Characteristically, in such a speculative gold rush a high proportion of the houses and offices have never been occupied. For their purchasers were not buying something which they intended to make use of themselves but a housing future. So, curiously, the 'New Town' of Docklands is a ghost town, its rush-built apartments not homes lived in by people who have any intention of developing local roots but corporate investments for visiting staff. Even those who move in are unlikely to stay more than a couple of years before they in turn make their killing. And some of the biggest blocks, for instance the 210,000 square-foot South Quay Plaza 3, have never been occupied.

The effects of this incubus have, despite the vivid

propaganda, been almost wholly negative. Far from creating local jobs, it has been the last straw for many firms. Some have been bought out at pre-LDDC prices by compulsory purchase. Others who might have survived if they could have expanded are out of the running at the new land price levels achieved by the speculators. The softwood trade, still important in the 1980s, was one of many which were forced out. Nor, predictably, have the new firms brought much work for East Enders. The new commercial firms bring their own staff with them. And the industrial incomers, notably the newspaper printers, were making the move as part of a massive shedding of staff anyway. The sort of jobs that did 'trickle down' were peripheral: cleaning, catering, guarding, selling hot dogs at the Arena, mopping the offices and manning the private security forces which roam the emptiness at night in pursuit of 'prowlers', people who lived there before the LDDC arrived. Even the vast construction programme has largely been carried out by migrant workers from the north of England, Ireland and Europe. The director of the London Docklands Local Purchasing Project, set up by the Canary Wharf developers Olympia & York and the LDDC specifically to encourage local recruitment, resigned in July 1990 in 'utter demoralisation', complaining of 'lack of co-operation, political gamesmanship and poor management'. A newspaper straw poll survey of twenty local building firms found only one had done any work at Canary Wharf or even been asked to tender. Although the Poplar Steam Baths was eventually turned into a training centre, it is not that easy to turn a docker or ship-repair worker into a steel erector overnight. It is said of the red brick road along Marsh Wall that not a single brick was laid by a local. Nor is there yet anywhere the building workers could afford to live if they chose, like the labourers who built the original docks, to stay. There is no Cubitt Town of the 1990s, just another block of luxury apartments called Curlew's something. If jobs do materialise eventually – and they will probably be pretty traditional, that is, menial: shelf-filling, cleaning up, portering – they will have been immensely expensive judged against the tremendous cost to the public exchequer of the LDDC as a whole.

Instead of a new sort of working community which has benefits for all emerging, the exact opposite has happened; a species of social apartheid. Islanders encountered the LDDC when it was taking away their communities, closing down local firms, buying up homes and cafés by compulsory purchase, shooing them off their imposing buildings and knocking down their homes to build motorways no-one wants. The fortified wall which had once circled the docks was not so much torn down as rearranged as a series of fences, barriers, security gates and keep-out signs which seek to keep the working class away from the new proletarian-free yuppie zones. A typical action is that of a group of high-income Dockneys (the yuppy Isle of Dogs residents' self-designation) who sued their private landowners because they failed to curb the 'nuisance' of the indigenous neighbours who had a propensity for shouting and hanging out washing. But few of the luxury residential developments have even got the degree of organisation to complain. Their owners are either subletting or absent most of the time in their weekend homes, or living invisibly behind high security in their refuge-with-a-view, insulated from anything outside the front door. Children, if there are any, are packed away at boarding school, health problems sorted out by private subscription, and groceries bought over the phone or computer. It is the future if the world was to be ruled by estate agents. And it doesn't work. And even had it wished to, the LDDC could have done little to redress the underfinancing of the NHS, the downgrading of employment benefit, the low morale of London schools, the stagnating traffic, the rising crime and the battered local government which have been the other side of the Thatcher coin which paid it so generously. But it could have made gestures in the boom years of the mid- and late 1980s when it had the income to do so rather than expressing good intentions when the boom was over and the money had run out or been spent on providing Canary Wharf with a motorway of its own.

The final irony is that those who live by speculation also die by it. The theory that new specialist office facilities, constructed with computerised dealing facilities designed in, could undercut office floorspace prices in the City of London's fast overcrowding square mile, was predicated on the City's deregulation in Big Bang. As Wayne Travelstead, the original developer of the Canary Wharf site, argued, every international bank and dealing house would now need its base in London and the traditional City couldn't cope. But not only has Black Monday imploded Big Bang and left many international firms licking their wounds, slimming their London staff and contemplating withdrawal, but the City itself has fought back. The City's lateral expansion at Broadgate and the Spitalfields Market site vastly increased its office space and stabilised prices. Fleet Street has been reshaped from a printing centre into housing for the financial market, and the City has even built upon itself, as in the giant office complex built astride the road at London Wall near the Barbican. The initial price attraction of the Isle of Dogs, with its primitive travel access and rudimentary local facilities, was, by the recession of the 1990s, looking distinctly less glittering and Canary Wharf's 12 million square feet of office space distinctly hard to let. 'In the next few years, one city will emerge to rival the world's leading business centres. With formidable financial trading power. A city where people will go to work on a £3 billion transport system' drooled the advertisements, concluding hopefully: 'It's not a famous city but it will be.' While the corridors of dog food and malls of toilet rolls at the pre-LDDC Asda remain well patronised by Island families getting on with life as best they can, the pricey specialist shops in Tobacco Dock do desultory trade with only thirty-six of its sixty units open. And the general collapse of the London property boom has been still more dramatic in Docklands with house prices remorselessly falling since 1989. Those who bought speculatively in the easy money days can't get rid of them and the frenzy which converted Victorian buildings into (often rather shoddy) 'luxury apartments' has left a lot of developers stuck with unsaleable assets. And upriver, Butler's Wharf can't sell enough flats to cover its interest charges.

This in turn has required a change in direction for the corporation. For eight years it boasted about its 'single-minded' lack of interest in the community it was usurping and its lack of liaison with the elected dockland local authorities. But under Michael Honey's chairmanship and some prodding from the Department of the Environment Select Committee, the line changed. In the 1990s, joint planning documents on health and welfare issues started to proliferate and funding for schemes which might benefit Islanders, still modest, replaced the previous stony indifference. And it became increasingly clear that, not least through the direct lobbying on transport exerted by the Canary Wharf developers, the fiction that Docklands was self-financed was over and massive (unplanned) public investment, on the developers' terms, was to be pumped into the project. One thus ends with the worst of both worlds in Docklands. The project has been enormously expensive to the public purse, yet much of the spending, such as the Canary Wharf Jubilee Line extension (£1,000 million, 90 per cent government-financed) and the Limehouse Link underground motorway (£240 million from the Department of Transport), doesn't make sense if the needs of London are considered as a whole. The depth of the 1990 recession has forced the LDDC to shelve its plans for renovation of the Royal Group of docks in Newham and put in jeopardy the social 'Accord' struck

with Tower Hamlets Council as the price for the Limehouse Link motorway.

The chances for Docklands developing into anything
that one could recognise as a city are remote, and there
is a real possibility that with the slump in the building
industry in Britain and continued high interest rates
hitting the big developers not just the luxury homes
but office developments will never be occupied. The
delay consequent on Mrs Thatcher's ambivalence
towards the EEC has probably fatally weakened London's chances of emerging as the premier centre of
European banking. The London City Airport has strug-
gled since it opened in October 1987; the Docklands
Light Railway, described in the LDDC's 87/88 Annual
Review as the 'cornerstone of the Corporation's commitment to increasing and improving public transport
in Docklands', is still shut at weekends and evenings;
and the Thamesline Riverbus (given £500,000 government aid in February 1989 to stave off collapse) remains
expensive and usually empty. By the end of 1990, both
Tobacco Dock and Terence Conran's Butler's Wharf
complex, two of the more architecturally interesting
developments, went into receivership. The existing
roads run at standstill speeds due to weight of traffic –
the Commercial Road regularly comes to a standstill
during peak hours – and all that has 'trickled down' is
gravel and slime from the excavation lorries.

If Canary Wharf were to survive the competition of
Broadgate, King's Cross and Croydon, solve its transportation problems and manage to fill up its vast floorspace, it might eventually prove profitable to its
owners. But still hellish for those who lived there in
the shadow of the tower blocks, which at night will be
as dead and demoralising as the Wall Street area of
Manhattan. It is, some might say cynically, simply the
oldest of city stories: the callous indifference to the
social consequences for the existing population in the
pursuit of profit. But when this process happened in
London in the late nineteenth century, it was moderated

by a sense of civic pride and social conscience and underwritten by an empire whose super-profits could afford acts of charity and municipal contrition. It is by now blindingly obvious that any large city depends on regulation, maintenance and investment by an elected authority to protect it from despoliation by landowners and commercial interests. It needs a logical transport system and adequate housing and sanitation if it is not to choke itself to death. We didn't know what happens when a national government declines to take responsibility for its capital city but we are beginning to find out: homelessness, crime, crashes, traffic jams taking place between towering rebuilds and revamps of commercial sites whose values rise remorselessly but whose 'streets' contain only the national retail chains who can afford the rents and commuters scurrying for their coaches home.

And even if it did work, it would surely be unacceptable for those whose labour over generations has created the astronomical value of central London land to be simply kicked off by those who hold the title to the sod. Yet small-scale industrial regeneration, artisan workshops, widening of green spaces, some measure of dwellers' control, to evolve a successor to large-scale manufacturing, is ruled out by the high interest rates, exorbitant rents and privatisation. And the Thatcher Government, and the commercial interests it so forcefully represented, was not just uninterested in but actively hostile to developments in this direction. Its animus against the GLC was not just ideological but economic, for as a regional strategic body it could be quite effective in alliance with local residential groups, as at Covent Garden, Coin Street, or Spitalfields, in legally halting or at least hampering the property developers.

Even if one accepted that there was no alternative to turning over inner London to private developers, those vested with planning authority could be quite versatile in imposing terms on them. The now elderly New

Town of Letchworth has operated a scheme since its onset whereby 50 per cent of the increase in land value is divided between owners and the New Town Corporation. But when a weakened version of such a scheme, only operative if the Canary Wharf developers moved into 'super-profit', was mooted by the LDDC's financial advisers, they meekly accepted that the first Canary Wharf was unsurprisingly 'not interested' in profit-sharing. And when the second Olympia & York consortium then took over the deal at a bargain basement price, they were even less interested in pursuing profit-sharing, despite the potentially enormous income from the complex. The LDDC had boxed themselves into Olympia & York, or else: 'What is to be remembered at the time was that there were no other organisations ready to consider the comprehensive development of Canary Wharf on the scale envisaged that would produce the kind of economic benefits which were judged to flow back from this scheme,' as Michael Honey put it to the House of Commons Committee on Public Accounts in 1988. A development corporation without direct accountability to the public or responsibility beyond selling off land to the highest bidder ends up hoist on its own petard, accepting offers with absolutely no civic, architectural, or community merit and putting a brave face on it. It then finds itself obliged to produce a roadlink which is immensely destructive to an established community, 'Limehouse Link', and a tube extension which contradicts the recommendations of all its transport advisers. This spineless approach even reneged on the specification for the UDCs which were proposed in the light of the New Town experience by the Town and Country Planning Association. They had specified that UDCs should 'only be set up within a particular inner city area if the local authority agrees', that they should produce 'agreed planning and development strategies for the whole of the urban areas in which they are located', that there should be an 'ongoing consultation process with the local people to determine their needs and wishes', and lastly that 'a small majority' of members should be drawn from local authorities for that area.

The tragedy is immense: Docklands was the world's choicest building site. Between the Royals and St Katherine's Dock, an area was freed for new use larger than the whole of the city of Venice. At the centre of a great capital was a chance to plan and design with vision. It didn't need to become a jumble lot of giant offices at the whim of land prices driven dizzy by speculation and recession. The possibilities were there. As the architectural critic Stephen Gardiner wrote before the LDDC took off: 'Land is no longer scarce and . . . the pressure on land values should be reduced. Moreover, if rents and building heights were limited . . . land values would also be limited. The dock area could be developed as a residential centre for Londoners at reasonable prices on one of the best sites in the world – overlooking the Thames.' Instead of what the architect Richard Rogers describes as 'a hymn to greed', Docklands could have evolved a mixture of commercial and residential building which on the Thames and facing Europe could have been an internationally minded inner city with perhaps a university and colleges, an artists' community and facilities for light manufacture, artisan work, studios, workshops and recreation. Professor Tony West, associated with the artists now driven and priced out of St Katherine's, was prescient in 1978: 'What is needed in Docklands is some freedom. Less efficiency is required at the top, more inefficiency – let people get on with their own lives, let them have the space to express themselves without harassment from above.'

Exactly the reverse has happened: the totalitarian obelisk of Canary Wharf dominates the area physically and politically, while on the muddy ground the various security firms move the locals on and the area is stifled by cars and lorries. The much-vaunted benefits brought by the LDDC are also exaggerated. First, the Department of the Environment funding to the LDDC, even when it results in direct grants towards housing, health and education, does little to counteract the reduction of central aid towards the provision of good-quality public services from the local authority. It is conscience money and spread thin at that. The new developments don't bring appropriate jobs into the borough because of a gross mismatch of skills. A skills gap was inevitable in any regeneration and could have been planned for, but the LDDC's approach made things much worse. Rates didn't increase the local council's purse straight-forwardly, since increased income was offset against central government subsidies to Docklands. And after the introduction of the poll tax and the uniform business rate, such income will be collected and spent nationally. Nor does the much vaunted Section 52, 'planning gain', always bring as much relief as hoped. It hasn't always arrived and obviously can only be spent on capital pro-jects.

Even very tangible apparent gains are double-edged. The Island may have got a cash machine at last, but shopping opportunities are not much enhanced for Islanders by luxury retailers in marble malls. And Michael Barraclough's successful self-build housing project, a true co-operative of skills and enterprise, is now worth so much due to land price inflation that there is immense pressure on the self-builders to cash in their hard-sweated chips and move to Essex.

The truth is plain. The commercial forces now want outcast E14 for themselves. The LDDC has executed a coup and installed a dictatorship with skilled financing and subtle PR rather than bullets and grenades. But the consequences are distinctly Latin American. Consul-tation, let alone local democracy, is given only lip ser-vice. Rather than a plan which fits the people, the LDDC have got rid of the people who don't fit the plan. Yet East Enders want to go on living in the East End, as was shown by the tenacity of the Bengalis in Spitalfields and the repudiation of the Housing Action

Trust schemes by tenants who were offered improvements their estates required only if they relinquished their security of tenure. The economic forces now levering apart existing communities in the East End are as powerful as and more dangerous than those unleashed in the Blitz or the benign incompetence of the first phase of postwar rebuilding.

But this conflict is sharpening the political consciousness of modern East Enders and giving new meanings to old lessons. Resistance *is* possible but in altered circumstances new tactics are required. The people of Limehouse could not stop the Limehouse Link and save the 500 homes which were demolished to clear a path for it. But tenants fought hard for transfer to accommodation of high quality and groups of neighbours often succeeded in moving *en bloc*. The tenants' association successfully insisted that a nearby luxury residential block be requisitioned for the 'decanting', and many Limehouse pensioners from the Barleycorn Estate now enjoy a view of scenic waterfalls and uniformed caretakers on the front entrance. Double glazing was, eventually, installed for those who stayed behind and when the noise was still excessive the tenants invaded the building site, once stopping the bulldozers for one and a half hours. Rank and file building workers from the Construction Safety Campaign have protested, successfully, against the big building corporations and picketed coroners' courts and safety inquiries. The steel erectors at Canary Wharf organised genuine trade unions and struck for eleven weeks for better wages. SPLASH (the South Poplar, Limehouse Action for Secure Housing) was formed by over 5,000 tenants who now live in the middle of Europe's biggest building site and, angry at being ignored by the LDDC, campaign actively for proper compensation, comprehensive renovation and the recovery of land and housing ceded to the developers so that those on the waiting list can be given hope. The tall masts of the sailing clippers are long gone and pine trunks are no longer hauled aboard

SOME LIVES!

at the Greenland Dock. But new political saplings are finding their way upward and through them a new, or perhaps very old, East End will be born.

CHAPTER 13

UNHAPPY CITY

By the end of Mrs Thatcher's eleven years of office, London had undergone a dramatic change in both its physical appearance and its economic character. Now enduring its inevitable downside of economic recession and property slump, we are only slowly realising the social costs and consequences of Thatcher's sado-monetarism. The 1980s, a decade of free market 'liberalism', privatisation and remorselessly rising property prices, generated a commercial building boom to house the Big Bang of deregulated dealing and screen-based trading. '*Si monumentum requiris*' look round from the monumental folly of Canary Wharf and see the humiliation of ordinary Londoners by the triumphal obelisks of commerce. But look too at the other linchpins of London's architectural identity: Piccadilly Circus, Soho, Liverpool Street Station and Waterloo Station, The Angel and Battersea Bridge, all remade in the Thatcher mould, newly clad in the gleaming impenetrable façades of modern North American commercial architecture with their antiseptic malls, sterile piazzas, ghostly galleria and glacial curtain walls.

And with the decline of existing council housing and the virtual halt on new public housing starts, traditional working-class residential areas like Fulham, Battersea, Islington and parts of the East End were recolonised by the middle classes. This process is highly unpopular but has proved impossible to resist. The abolition of the Greater London Council and the underfinancing and undermining of inner London councils, together with the general decline in the NHS, education and welfare services, makes it very difficult for working-class Londoners effectively to oppose the process. Halting London's loss of manufacture or reversing land ownership patterns is a tall order when you are struggling to stump up the poll tax, waiting in pain for an elusive hospital bed, or looking after the children at short notice because there are not enough teachers that day.

So the reshaping of our metropolis is experienced passively in odd disjointed glimpses: the grimness of a once excellent public transport service stuck in semipermanent traffic jams, the thundering skip lorries, helmets, grit and strange shantytown feeling of ubiquitous rebuilding, being begged from by fit young people in theatre doorways, the sudden flash of riot among Nelson's lions. But in a way it's not surprising that the price of a re-creation of 'Victorian values' to our most Victorian of cities should be a dirty, lawless, polluted capital where the very rich spend much of their time protecting their wealth from an increasingly disaffected and disenfranchised working class. And the respectable middle class despair of both and concentrate on the struggle to keep the aspidistra flying by paying up their credit cards promptly. This sort of polarisation has after all happened before and led, in London, to the upsurges in the mid-nineteenth century which brought about the Reform Bill, to the post First World War agitation (known as 'Poplarism') which led to the richer boroughs assisting the poor in housing and welfare, and to the work of the interwar LCC and the postwar Labour Government's 'Welfare State'.

But late twentieth-century restructuring of inner London means something more fundamental than a lot of Lego-like office blocks and the return of the braying classes to Soho dining rooms. It requires the ejection of the urban proletariat and tradespeople from the city centre. The traditional London pattern of flat residential villages arranged on centuries-old road and river networks, a topography retained in this century by the emplacements and groynes of low-rent council housing which shielded the human heart of the city, is changing rapidly. Canary Wharf and the LDDC are only the most ostentatious example of a process by which multinational commercial developers, largely financed and controlled from outside Britain, will have been allowed to create a new 'free market' metropolis much more like an American city built from scratch in this century and dominated by a series of monocomplexes of offices, roads, national retail chains and leisure centres. The particular street plan of London allowed its intimate, artisan, unhurried qualities and logical patterns to its workshops, pubs, churches and houses. But these *quartiers populaires* are disappearing, declared inconvenient to the free working of the internal combustion engine and the market.

The immovable parts of nineteenth-century London like its museums, art galleries and great public buildings will be increasingly isolated from day-to-day life and scholarship and be utilised for ceremony and tourism. Londoners may man the booths, sweep the steps and guard the treasures but the visitors will be Americans and Japanese. The British Museum and the V and A will no longer be, as they were intended, a source of education and wonder to the citizens of London but instead just another nodal point on the printed circuits of international tourism. The life of the streets (which requires first streets and then people who live and work and grow up in them) has been the consistent source of London's vivacity and urbanity whether pictured by Hogarth, Eliot or MacInnes. Yet it too is being extinguished by crime, cars and the other unwanted side effects of this business-led redevelopment. In a real sense, citizens of London have been living in a conquered city; psychologically sacked, its democracy abolished, its assets sold off, its municipal pride humiliated, subject to intermittent disasters and terrifying shows of state force. We are not yet as far down the decivilisation process as Manhattan but increasingly the experience of living in this city is of being a victim of its random cruelty and lack of human scale.

'The inner cities next,' announced Mrs Thatcher in her 1987 paroxysm of third-term triumph in 1987: what she meant was the recolonisation of the old proletarian-bohemian, artisanal-shopkeeping, Labour-voting areas of the city centre by the values and the personnel of the Home Counties. In that process the proletarians, especially those among them who are poor, socially unattractive, sick or mentally ill are debarred from both production and consumption. There are jobs, minus tiresome, old-fashioned things like unions, closing times and safety regulations, as cooks and nannies, waiters and drivers, cleaners and guards, entertainers and prostitutes: jobs Londoners have always done by choice but are now expected, like cheerful imbeciles, to delight in or else. But very little production in the great manufacturing districts which once shaped London's industrial physiognomy: the light engineering of North-West London, the newspaper printing of Fleet Street, the docks- and river-related industries of the East End, the furniture and shoe workplaces of Hackney and Shoreditch. Ordinary Londoners, whose parents and grandparents built the capital and created its wealth, are increasingly in the way. Expensively in the way, consumers of the wrong things: not high-priced leisure products but hospitals, schools and social services.

There are precise parallels to late nineteenth-century London when a much more successful British capitalism's *laissez-faire* approach to social issues was breaking down round its ears with the impoverished fighting the police and looting in affluent central London while the rich complained of a 'plague of beggars' and the 'demoralised residuum'. Then the working-class quarters and the ungovernable rookeries of the poor were simply abolished by the great highways and sanitation schemes driven through by architects like Bazalgette. A century later the process is less brutal: the in-the-ways are bought out rather than thrown out. The immigrants who scrimped and saved to buy their own home but now have low and falling real incomes are persuaded to realise the raised value of their house and move to the suburbs. The public housing sector shrinks further when people who have exercised their 'right to buy' in turn sell out. And if growing children manage to find their way into council housing of their own by becoming parents then they push the homeless, the overcrowded and the student still further back in the ever-extending queue for a diminishing housing stock. London-wide, we have the threats to destroy homes and parks to provide more spaces for traffic jams, the lowest level of public expenditure on transport in Europe and mile after mile of dispiriting, indistinguishable high streets with their fast food franchises, boutique chains and video stores. Bernard Shaw, who was turned into a socialist by the social and economic chaos and cruelty of late nineteenth-century London, wrote over a hundred years ago that what the city needed was 'the development of individual greed into civic spirit; of the extension of the laissez-faire principle to public as well as private enterprise; of bringing all the citizens to a common date in civilisation'. Architectural facelifts would be of no value 'until London belongs to, and is governed by, the people who use it'.

The despoliation of our cities concerns me not just as a Londoner but as a doctor because it generates a great deal of ill-health, depression and family disruption. It is compounded by the reversal over the same decade of the century-long trend towards greater equality of income and the prising open of the already wide gap between the rich and poor. The consequences of that economic process are presented in human terms, conveniently out of sight to the politicians, in our surgeries every day. Patients made sick by poverty, living an unhealthy, overcrowded existence which is exhausting them and making them ill. Mrs Thatcher's chosen monument may be the commercial majesty of Canary Wharf topped out only two weeks before her resignation in November 1990, but I see the social cost which has been paid for it in the streets of the East End: the schizophrenic dementing in public, the young mother bathing the newborn in the sink of a B-and-B, the pensioner dying pinched and cold in a decrepit council flat, the bright young kids who can get dope much easier than education, wasted on smack. I also see the pain of those trying to cope in the social services whose collective provision the Thatcher era systematically derided, underfinanced and then 'reformed': the student nurse reduced to tears trying to manage a night-time surgical ward singlehanded, the infant school teachers improvising multicultural assemblies with jungles made of donated coloured paper while their children's outside lavatories rot and the cleaning ladies don't get their wages, the social workers who break down in surgery grey with exhaustion and despair. These were the years when hospital after hospital was boarded up in the East End and the Prime Minister told us the health service 'was safe in her hands' while waltzing off to private hospitals when she got ill. It was the decade when waiting lists lengthened and our patients were sent home from hospital ill and in pain while the minister stated, 'I do not accept that the NHS is underfunded. Why do we go through the rigmarole of dusting off the same stories every year?' It was the decade when the NHS, a triumphant example of the superiority of collective action and public initiative in an area where the 'law of the market' is seen at its worst, was forced into decline and disorganisation.

I see the consequences in my own colleagues who however hard they work cannot substitute for the accelerating closures and lengthening waiting lists in the hospital service which arise specifically from hasty, ill-thought-out and illogical government market-imitating

234

measures. For GPs themselves have had imposed a new contract which has profoundly changed and deeply demoralised a profession whose morale was previously high. Again I see a sequence of faces: the cowed, apologetic face of the BMA's negotiator facing ninety hostile East London GPs; the beefy fury of a Kensington GP firebrand at a delegates meeting in an airless lecture theatre in Bloomsbury ranting at 'Quisling negotiators'; a new general manager in the ornate boardroom of the local psychiatric hospital disintegrating into incoherence as he attempted to explain how his hospital 'opting out' would improve health care in the locality. Predictably GPs' indignation at being subjected to a middle-class productivity deal didn't impel them to working-class-type trade union organisation to protect their own conditions of work and wages. Instead after all the hot air we ended up obediently filling in the forms and endlessly correcting statistics in a paper chase which required considerable extra work, little extra resources and a probable worsening of quality of the overall standards of patient care.

What has happened instead was perhaps more profound, the ideological defection of a profession which was overwhelmingly Conservative in party loyalty and political outlook. What they have experienced is a microcosm of the Thatcher years no less than Canary Wharf. It is a process of decivilisation in which what doctors prided as a personal relationship between themselves and the patient, is now reshaped by the commodity-process. Instead of an overall income derived from providing, according to their own judgement, appropriate general medical care, income becomes, as it was pre-NHS, increasingly derived from individual items of service as they are carried out on individual persons in competition with one's erstwhile colleagues. Prevention for populations, service according to need, the family doctors' very idea of themselves as people who had time to grieve with their patients, to share the joy of childbirth, the crisis of illness and the time of

day in the corner shop, are swept away. The New
Model GP is hunched over the computer screen calculating uptake and turnover, auditing not clinical skill
but fiscal returns and acting as an accountant, an architect, a travel agent, a manager: almost anything but a
doctor.

What is happening to the human relationships
between GP and patient is a part of the same process
which is making the quality of life so much worse for
the urban have-nots: the old, the jobless, the overcrowded, the giro-dependent. Just as the ripping asun-
der of Limehouse by the LDDC is part of the same
process that created Cardboard City and emptied
County Hall. And what is being lost is something infinitely precious, that sense of neighbourhood, community and mutual solidarity which has given London
its special character. People are a city, populations
allowed some stability to grow and work and educate
themselves. This cannot be achieved on unmaintained
dump estates where eye contact can be risky, it's
dangerous to talk to a neighbour and everyone wants
out. Or when the civic authorities are debarred from
undertaking anything but the most basic of collective
provision for municipal well-being. It can't be created
when schools and hospitals and housing are neglected and
nurses, teachers and architects constantly demeaned.
It cannot be done, as the LDDC experience shows so
devastatingly, by abandoning planning and letting
'market forces' rip. We need to have done with an
era when 'community', as in 'community charge' or
'community care', was a dirty word. We need to plan
again, to protect the wide mixtures of land use which
would make our city healthy once more. We need to
recover for the citizens of London some real freedom
and genuine choice. We need to recover from the developers and the estate agents' thrall different and better
possibilities: of low-rent housing, smaller-scale manufacture, informal places and unofficial uses. We have to
stop showering hardship on the working class of the

inner cities and instead respect their ingenuity, their bravery and their beauty. For the true makers of a city are not those who possess its property statutes but those who live there. And when they are forced out of their homes and when their lives are made impossible by a government which has contempt for them, London will have lost not only its human identity but its very soul. The East End was never grand but it had what Mildred Rose calls 'a style of living that was coherent and lustily alive'. It deserves to get it back.

BIBLIOGRAPHY

Caroline Adams
  Across Seven Seas and Thirteen Rivers:
  Life Stories of Pioneer Sylhetti Settlers in Britain
  THAP Books. London. 1987.
Bethnal Green and Stepney Trades Council
  Blood on the Streets
  London. 1978.
Simon Blumenfeld
  Jew Boy
  Lawrence and Wishart. London. 1986.
Toby Buxton
  Off Our Backs: The State of Industry and Employment in
  Tower Hamlets
  Tower Hamlets Information Research and Resource
Centre. London. 1986.
  A Second Look: a photographic record of a walk through Hack-
  ney in the 1890s and today
  Centerprise. London. 1975.
Department of Community Medicine, Tower Hamlets
Health Authority
  Tower Hamlets People
  London. 1989.
Docklands Consultative Committee
  Urban Development Corporations: Six Years in London's
  Docklands
  London. 1988.

BIBLIOGRAPHY

Kerry Downes
Hawksmoor
Thames and Hudson. London. 1970.
William J. Fishman
East End Jewish Radicals 1875–1914
Duckworth. London. 1975.
East End 1888
Duckworth. London. 1988.
William J. Fishman and Nicholas Breach
The Streets of East London
Duckworth. London. 1980.
William J. Fishman, Nicholas Breach, John M. Hall
East End and Docklands
Duckworth. London. 1990.
Charlie Forman
Spitalfields, a Battle for Land
Hilary Shipman. London. 1989.
Bernard Gainer
The Alien Invasion: The origins of the Aliens Act of 1905
Heinemann. London. 1972.
Mark Girouard, Dan Cruickshank, Raphael Samuel et al.
The Saving of Spitalfields
Spitalfields Historic Building Trust. London. 1989.
Gina Glasman
East End Synagogues
Museum of the Jewish East End. London. 1987.
Greater London Council
The East End File
London. 1983.
Paul Harrison
Inside the Inner City
Penguin. Harmondsworth. 1983.
David Harvey
The Urban Experience
Blackwell. Oxford. 1989.
Dick Hobbs
Doing The Business: Entrepreneurship, the Working Class and Detectives in the East End of London
Clarendon Press. Oxford. 1988.
Eve Hostettler (ed.)
The Island at War: Memories of War-time Life on the Isle of Dogs
Island History Trust. London.

House of Commons Committee of Public Accounts
  20th Report. *On Urban Development Corporations*
  HMSO. London. 1989.
House of Commons Home Affairs Committee
  1st Report. *Bangladeshis in Britain*
  HMSO. London. 1986.
Colm Kerrigan
  A History of Tower Hamlets
  London Borough of Tower Hamlets. Libraries Department. 1982.
Joanna Mack and Steve Humphries
  London at War
  Sidgwick and Jackson. London. 1985.
Peter Marcan
  Artists and the East End
  Peter Marcan Publications. High Wycombe. 1986.
Frank Martin
  Rogues' River
  Ian Henry Publications. Hornchurch. 1983.
Henry Mayhew
  Mayhew's London
  Edited by Peter Quennell. Bracken Books. London. 1984.
Albert Meltzer
  The Anarchists in London 1935–1955
  Cienfuegos Press. Orkney Islands. 1976.
Findlay Muirhead
  London and its Environs
  Macmillan/Hachette. London/Paris. 1922.
Museum of London
  The Quiet Conquest: The Huguenots 1685–1985
  London. 1985.
Ian Nairn
  Nairn's London
  Penguin. Harmondsworth. 1966.
Alan Palmer
  The East End: Four Centuries of London Life
  John Murray. London. 1989.
John Pearson
  The Profession of Violence
  Panther. London. 1973.
John Pender and Paul Wallace
  The Square Mile

BIBLIOGRAPHY

Nikolaus Pevsner
The Buildings of England. London (except the cities of London and Westminster
Penguin. Harmondsworth. 1952.

Tony Phillips
A London Docklands Guide
Peter Marcan Publications. High Wycombe. 1986.

Tony Phillips
The Pubs of Tower Hamlets
London Borough of Tower Hamlets. Libraries Department. London. 1988.

John Pudney
London's Docks
Thames and Hudson. London. 1975.

Steen Eiler Rasmussen
London, The Unique City
Pelican. Harmondsworth. 1960.

Mildred Rose
The East End of London
Cresset Press. London. 1951.

Aumie and Michael Shapiro
The Jewish East End: More Memories
Springboard. London. 1987.

A. G. Thompson
The Romance of London River
Bradley and Son Ltd. London. 1934.

Rozina Visram
Ayahs, Lascars and Princes
Pluto Press. London. 1986.

Colin Ward
Welcome Thinner City: Urban Survival in the 1990s
Bedford Square Press. London. 1989.

David Widgery
Beating Time. Riot'n'Race'n'Rock'n'Roll
Chatto. London. 1986.

Elizabeth and Wayland Young
London Churches
Grafton. London. 1986.

Sharon Zukin
Loft Living. Culture and Capital in Urban Change
Radius. London. 1988.

INDEX

242

INDEX

243

INDEX

INDEX

246

INDEX

and children, 109
as cause of ill-health, 115, 233
growth of, 108
increase of, 114
pregnancy, 25, 44, 50–1, 54, 56, 57, 65, 90, 101, 113, 115, 117, 152, 162
as grounds for dismissal, 88
prescription charges, increased, 25
Princes Lodge, 14, 116, 119
prison, 24, 86, 105, 118, 142, 147
privacy, lack of, 74, 108
privatisation, 111
property market, collapse of, 41, 221
prostitutes, 46, 232
prostitution, 7, 94, 105, 114, 115, 142
Providence Row night shelter, 119
Psychiatric Intensive Therapy Unit, 148
psychogeriatric care, 129, 130
psychotic illness, 150
pubs, 73, 101, 140
puerperal psychosis, 23
Punjabis, 171

racism, 186
rape, 7, 16, 52, 82, 84, 105, 153, 174
in the family, 85
Rasul, Syed, 205
Ratcliff, 172
recession, 159
redundancy, 21
Reichmann, Mr, 169
rent arrears, 113
rents, as percentage of income, 118
republicanism, Irish, 193
respiratory problems, 75, 80, 115, 204
Ridley Road market, 38
right-to-buy schemes, 117
River Lea, 30, 33, 35
River Thames, 33, 35, 40, 91, 207–28
Riverbus, 222
road accidents, 157
Rock Against Racism, 204
Rocker, Fermin, 188
Rocker, Rudolph, 188–9, 205
Rocque, John, 177
Rogers, Richard, 225
Roman Road market, 38
Rose, Mildred, 237
Rosewarne, David, 37
Rotherhithe Tunnel, 172
Royal Commission on Alien Immigration, 191
runaway teenagers, 115
Russia, 184
Russian Revolution, 190
Russians, 185, 186

Salmon and Ball pub, 178
Salvation Army, 14, 99, 116, 119, 139
Samuel Lewis Trust, 35
sanitary towels, allergy to, 22
Savage, Wendy, 87
scabies, 92
schizophrenia, 17, 139
school admission, 88
school meals, 69
school milk, free, 62
school-leavers, 44, 45, 67
schools, 219, 232
Scott, Ronnie, 182
Scurr, John, 89
seamen, 175, 189, 194, 196, 198, 211

Bengali, 199–200
lodgings for, 116
seaside, 72
council trips to, 128
sex, unsafe, 147
sex education, 52
sexual antagonism between men and women, 86
sexual relationships, 86, 94
Shaw, George Bernard, 188, 233
ship repair industry, 42
shipbuilding, 208
shoe-makers, 30
shoe-making industry, 31, 232
shoes, as indicator of income, 111
shop stewards' committees, in docks, 213
shoplifting, 114
sick notes, 44
Sikhs, 91, 151
silk looms, breaking of, 179
Silvertown, 33, 34, 42
single mothers, 53, 85, 117, 123
single parents, 14, 85–6, 114
single-parent families, 174
Skid Row, 139–51
slavery, 197–8
slaves, freed, 197
sleeping rough, 120
Smith, Sam, 192, 193
smoking, 2, 62, 70, 73, 75, 76, 79, 90, 96, 99, 106, 112–13, 122, 142, 162
Social Fund loans, 115
social security, 19, 85
social workers, 234
socialism, 16, 74, 187, 188
solidarity: East End, 16
in everyday life, 74
trade union, 190
Somalia, 174
Somalis, 14, 105, 153, 196
Somers, Freddy, 192
Sorges family, 137
soup kitchens, 187
South Poplar, Limehouse Action for Secure Housing (SPLASH), 227
South Quay Plaza, 162, 217
Spaniards, 174
special needs education, 158
speculation, property, 220
Spitalfields, 31, 172, 174, 177, 178, 179, 187, 212, 220, 223, 226
squatters, 99, 101, 204
squatting movement, 147, 191
St Anne's church, Limehouse, 12, 14, 33, 172
St George's in the East church, 33, 186
St Joseph's church, 193
St Mary le Bow church, 29
Stepney, 31, 34, 172, 190, 191, 212
steroids, use of, 78
still birth, 52, 53, 115
stonemasons, 46
Stracey, John H., 6
strikes, 191, 192
in clothing industry, 188–9
in docks, 190, 205
matchgirls, 40
strokes, 125, 126
suicide, 85, 103, 135
among unemployed, 123
swearing, 4
'sweating' system, 43

INDEX

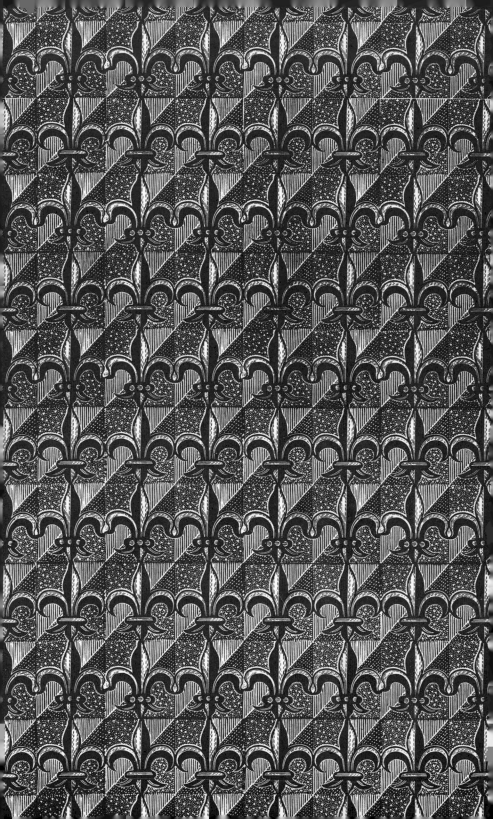